NATIVE AMERICAN HERBAL REMEDIES AND HERBAL RECIPES

Bimala Goel

Table of Contents

INTRODUCTION

The Native American people used diverse techniques for curing and caring for their bodies. They had a multitude of herbal remedies as well as massage, sweating, and steam as some examples. One such herbal remedy is the dandelion root to cure an upset stomach. This book will explore how these people use herbs in their daily lives.

Different types of plants were used for medicinal purposes throughout Native American history. Some were employed for making medicine, some to cure a skin ailment, and others as a meal. Animals and bodily fluids were a resource to heal other body parts. Most of these plants did not have the same effect on different people. One person may have a stronger reaction to a plant, while another may not notice any change in their health. What made some people feel better may not work for others either. Not all plants worked in the same way.

Native Americans used diverse methods for using their plants as a therapeutic remedy for various conditions that plagued them. Many of these healers used several native plants and different herbal remedies when facing an ailment or disease. Some of these remedies were made from mint, barberry, and many other herbs, while others were made from more recognizable herbs such as opium poppy. These remedies varied depending on the ailment those treating it suffered, but one herb was used repeatedly throughout history to cure any diseases. This herb was the dandelion.

Millions of people have used the dandelion for different

reasons in many forms throughout history. There are hundreds of diverse types of uses for dandelion, in addition to a multitude of medical benefits. Dandelions are also considered a weed, as they grow about everywhere. They have medicinal properties as well as culinary uses, and nutritional value.

Native Americans used the dandelion root and flower in many ways, one being simply a meal. For example, one Native American account describes how the Iroquois settled to enjoy some bread made from ground dandelions culled from the sides of the road around 1650. The bread was toasted and then spread with game butter, sometimes from the fat of squirrels roasted in a small fire before grinding up.

By the 18th century, milk and eggs were used as ingredients in dishes like this. The milk came from Native American cows bred for this purpose. The dandelion was boiled with the milk until it was an even consistency, then it was poured into a vat where it hardened and turned yellow like rich yellow cheese. The dandelion blossoms were gathered throughout the growing season and added to the mixture with fresh eggs beaten with butter to cook evenly inside the cheese while they aged on top of it.

The settlers also used dandelion to make wine. The plant was grown and pressed, then left to ferment. The wine occasionally included other local plants that created a more fruity and less bitter taste. Wild grape vines growing among the dandelions would lend a sweeter taste to these wines. Still, this practice infected the native grapes with an invasive virus that has even caused millions of dollars in damage to the local industry.

The people believed to have first taught the settlers about dandelions were known as "Pilgrims." The recipe for how they prepared their Dandelion Wine can be read in numerous books written about Pilgrim traditions. The Pilgrims would make their wine from the greens and flowers of dandelions. The leaves would be boiled in water until the liquid reached a syrupy consistency. The cooked leaves were then mixed into a barrel of red and white wine, creating an even more flavorful drink.

Native Americans used dandelion in many ways for medicinal purposes as well as for culinary reasons. This herb was also used to make decorations by the Native Americans, that created dolls out of it and other books, as well as what is known today as Indian Beads.

AN OVERVIEW OF NATIVE AMERICAN HERBS

Native American Medicine History

There is evidence of Native Americans healing each other from at least 1800 BCE. Evidence suggests that many healers used whole plant remedies and some animal parts. However, there is also a history of catching and drying herbs for use in the future. Many treatments used little or no processing.

Native Americans treated diseases differently than European settlers; these treatments followed different principles than we do today. One consequence was that it became difficult to establish a standard of care among groups, making it difficult for doctors who came to live with the tribe and treat its members. This resulted in short-term solutions being used to address long- term problems—sometimes with disastrous results. Another problem was that medicines were not tested consistently to ensure safety; therefore, many Native American remedies still contain unknown and possibly dangerous chemicals.

The Treatment Approach

Native American medicine is a complete framework that balances every sphere of our lives, including lifestyle and social interactions with our inner world. Native medicine assumes that the roots of every imbalance lie in the divine realm. During every recovery procedure, spiritual approaches are vital.

Including fees and rates, clinical guidelines are often clearly and uniquely tailored for the patient. They require, as part of the healing method, the process of fee negotiation. The Healing Elder seems to have the most healing strength, and the elder practitioner loses his prestige as a powerful healer when treatment fails. The person needing healing makes a proposition to the medical doctor and waits to see if it is approved. They rarely negotiate face- to-face. The customer leaves the bid outside the healer's door, and if it remains there till the morning, it means that it has not been approved, and they can go somewhere. Once they understand, therapy will, for example, start with a behavioral prescription, a pledge, a selfless act, genuine repentance, or scaling a holy mountain. Techniques include self-inquiry and discovery to ascertain whether there is a need for a dietary improvement, prayer, herbs, massage, a sweat lodge ritual, or a vision quest.

Theories

The main objective is to alter the patient's comprehension of the world through a healthier self-concept, increased acceptance of others, and behavior adjustments. The healer's goal is not only to treat sickness but to change the patient's overall approach towards life and the world around him. Native American medicine combines science as well as spirit with the onset of new technology. They mostly use herbal interventions and pharmaceuticals. We can explain this by narrating a Native American story on the use of herbal medicine. Barb, a wife, mother, and lawyer, is still fighting breast cancer. She did what she could normally do, and cancer continued to spread despite all her efforts. She met with an Indian elder named Big Nose in a sweat lodge. He wanted to understand what she was doing or what hadn't changed in her life. Deep inside, as a mother-wife and lawyer, she thought she was a loser, and now she's healing herself. It was the pessimistic self-talk that needed to end, Big Nose told her. Barb decided to let go of her arrogant thought that she would be cured and started to enjoy the moment with her family due to this relationship. Another story talks of a woman who had had extreme arthritis. She was desperately looking for the right healer. To facilitate recovery, physicians go beyond the current problem and understand that radical improvement is often required. The shifts are primary, herbs are secondary, and massage and prayer. Right relationships, the correction of relationships with ourselves, families, members of the society, and the spiritual environment are all effects of disruption of relationships and disease development.

Training

Native American healers, through apprenticeships, educate their students. For preparation, several weeks of testing the purpose and dedication of a student are vital. An apprentice gains patience and respect and acquires knowledge. Native medicine is still an oral tradition. It cannot be taught in an academic setting. Students may learn the skills required only by experience, and only when the learner is ready does the older instructor encourage them to begin a medical practice.

The Main Role of Ceremonies

A crucial aspect of traditional aboriginal healing is the ritual. Due to the close relationship between physical and spiritual well-being, body and soul should heal together. Popular healing rituals encourage well-being by representing traditional concepts of the world, creator, and spirit. Prayer, drumming, chants, poems, legends, and the use of several religious artifacts may be part of them. Wherever an ill person requires curing, healers can perform ceremonies, but the rituals are sometimes carried out in sacred places. The unique buildings are also mentioned as the Medicine Lodges for healing. Traditional healing services are considered holy wherever they occur and are only performed by the native healers and local spiritual facilitators. The Non-natives can take part only by invitation. Native powwows, on the other hand, have grown today into most social and cultural activities that include indigenous music, singing, drumming, regalia, and food. Most powwows welcome all persons.

The Medicine Wheel and the Four Directions

The Medicine Wheel, also called the Holy Hoop, has been used for health and healing by thousands of diverse Native American tribes. Also, Father Heaven, Spirit Tree, and Mother Earth represent the Four Paths, symbolizing the dimensions of well-being and life cycles. The Medicine Wheel could take several different shapes. It could be artwork, or an actual structure on the ground, such as an artifact or painting. Hundreds of thousands, if not millions, of medicine wheels have been built on tribal territories across North America in recent decades.

Meanings of the Four Directions

Medicine Wheel is viewed differently by various tribes.

Usually, each of the Four Directions (West, East, North, and South) is represented by a distinctive hue, such as red, black, yellow, and white, representing human races for some. The Directions may also indicate:

- Stages of life: birth, youth, adulthood (or elder), and death.
- Elements of nature: sun (or fire), water, earth, and air.
- Animals, bears, eagles, buffalo, wolves, and many more.
- Life's spiritual, emotional, intellectual, and physical dimensions.
- Spiritual, emotional, intellectual, and bodily aspects of life.
- Ceremonial plants, sweetgrass, tobacco, cedar, sage.

Healing Plants

Here are several plants used for healing and their possible uses.

- Pennyroyal: Pennyroyal is a mint-scented, invasive weed that can poison you if consumed in large quantities and, in some cases, is fatal. It's been used in herbal therapy to treat various diseases, such as discomfort, fever, and allergy symptoms. It also has insecticidal effects and, when coupled with other herbs like lemon balm or lavender oil, can be an excellent treatment for scabies or lice.
- Rosemary: Rosemary is a perennial herb with medicinal uses, such as alleviating joint pains when applied topically and treating digestive problems

when consumed internally. It comes from the mint family, along with other plants that are also used for medicine, including mint, eucalyptus, basil, oregano, etc.

- Yarrow: Yarrow is a perennial herb that grows throughout Europe and the United States. It has been used to treat wounds because of its antiseptic properties. The traditional use, for this reason, is to put the fresh plant directly on a wound to seal it shut or wrap it in cloth soaked in yarrow tea, which is made by boiling fresh yarrow leaves for a few minutes and drinking it while still hot.
- Cayenne: Cayenne is a perennial herb that grows in warm climates worldwide. It has many medicinal uses; it can be used internally or externally. Internally, cayenne can be consumed to treat joint pain, indigestion, stomach ulcers, and high cholesterol when consumed raw or mixed into certain foods such as eggs or salad dressing. It can also be taken as a capsule or swallowed in powder form. Externally, cayenne can be applied topically to treat pain, reduce swelling, and speed up the healing process. Some people put it directly on their skin (blended into a lotion or used with ointment), while others boil it in a pan of water and then use a towel to soak up the tea and rub it on the area where they are experiencing pain.
- Plantain: Plantain is a perennial herb that grows all over the world. It has been used as a medicinal herb for centuries, easing aches and pains when brewing tea.
- Burdock: Burdock is a perennial herb that grows all over the world. Its root has many medicinal

properties; it can be eaten raw or cooked (with other herbs), drunk as tea, infused into bath water, or applied topically. It has also been used in China to treat high blood pressure.

- Holy basil: Holy basil is a perennial herb that grows worldwide. It has long been used in India for medicinal purposes, aiding digestion, relieving diarrhea, and treating eye problems when brewed as herbal tea.

- Agrimony: Agrimony is a perennial herb that grows throughout Europe and much of Asia. It's been used for centuries as a remedy for palpitations and paleness of skin, including for those who have leprosy or have had their skin removed from them due to the infection caused by the disease.

- Comfrey: Comfrey is a perennial herb that grows all over the world. It can be eaten in many forms, either cooked or raw. It also has many medicinal properties, including treating wounds and easing arthritis pain because of its anti-inflammatory properties.

Intersections of Traditional and Western Healing

Today, the issue of either depending on conventional native healing practices or pursuing Western medical care is frequently confronted by Native Americans of both groups. The two cultures existed in coexistence relatively until recently, with no intersections between them. However, now, the continuum of health services can be accessed by Native Americans. Within tribal communities, most traditional healers are still practicing independently. To organize treatment for Native American patients, other healers can collaborate with Western-trained foremost care physicians. Some healthcare facilities, often at the exact location, provide both conventional and Western medicine. In certain areas, rather than by tribal health centers or hospitals, patients of Native Americans receive traditional healing from inside the local tribal population. In the Upper Plains Tribes of Lakota and Dakota, and Mandan, Hidatsa, and Arikara (MHA), tribal members arrange for the services by directly calling nearby healers. Many Western-trained doctors often recommend patients to conventional healers and may sometimes assist a specific patient in coordinating traditional and Western medicine.

NATIVE AMERICAN FORAGING RITUALS

As changes in the natural environment have threatened indigenous practices and led to significant cultural shifts, some tribes re- embraced their ancient foraging rituals.

For instance, the Southwest Indians of Arizona rely on women's rights to ensure a healthy harvest.

For other tribes, like those in Oaxaca, Mexico, whose subsistence depends on corn and beans, foraging is about more than just nourishment. The plants they collect hold the wisdom of centuries past, which they must keep alive to survive.

In this, we explore how Native American tribes adapt traditional foraging rituals to connect meaningfully with themselves and their land.

I'll present stories about foraging rites from Native peoples throughout North America in the following paragraphs. These rituals are essential for the traditions they represent and serve as a reminder that one of the most effective ways to restore ourselves and our environment is by reconnecting with nature and putting our best survival skills to work.

We'll start our journey by looking at ancient foraging rituals from early southwestern tribes like the Navajo and Hopi to ensure a fruitful harvest. And we'll finish by looking at how women in Oaxaca, Mexico, feel at home amongtheir corn, beans, and squash.

Ancient Foraging Rituals

Through the Southwest, most native foraging rituals were carried out by women. For example, before a Hopi woman or girl could eat Bitterroot (the plant from which they made their blue-black dye), she had to spend four days in seclusion and fast. She was forbidden from eating or drinking and couldn't leave her sleeping place until sunrise on the fourth day when her mother would ceremonially bathe her. Afterward, she would plant a seed of corn to show gratitudefor its gifts.

The Navajo also had many sacred rituals associated with hunting, gathering, and preparing food. First, there was a ceremony to rid the holy mountains of their jagged edges and smooth them. Then the hunter would ceremoniously make his first kill and offer it to Mother Earth. Finally, the tribe would strictly protect this animal for three days until his family members could take turns eating its flesh.

In Oaxaca, people come together with their corn, beans, and squash in a process called "masa" that connects them to their land and one another. The "maseca" is a ritual that ties all these elements together as relatives who work together on behalf of future generations.

"Masa" means "becoming linked, forming a bond, sowing seeds." The ritual is like a ceremony; people, crops, and animals are brought together. The tradition has changed in Oaxacan communities and south-central Mexico with a growing population and shifting agricultural practices. The growers participating in the current Masa among their neighbors have typically moved from two rustic family farms to small commercial farm units. And instead of using peyotes as part of their ceremonial medicine, they predominantly used grains such as corn and beans, which were once reserved for livestock feed.

As in many indigenous cultures, this toil is integral to Oaxacan life. And the maseca ritual helps farmers recognize this connection between their labor and the earth in a meaningful way. It's about showing appreciation for crops and food, ultimately helping keep the sacred traditions alive for future generations.

The process begins with a group of women who gather in each other's homes to begin the masa ritual seven days before the mazorca (corn) harvest is complete. The women bring individual portions of their harvest from home, but they also get corn from their neighbor's fields so that all parties are equally responsible for successful crop yields.

The women gather to prepare and cook an offering for the goddess of corn. Over a small fire, they make a heart-shaped offering in an earthenware pot. Next, they add sprouted corn seeds, beans, and squash—the "masa" or "seeds." The cooked masa is then eaten by everyone involved in the ritual while each person says a blessing over their food. The pattern is about making offerings to the goddess of corn and connecting farmers with one another through food sharing.

The seven days of the maseca ritual also allow time for helping neighbors bring their harvest home from their fields. All those involved in the masa ritual know the importance of preserving the sacred tradition that connects them to their land and future generations.

The maseca ritual is also an opportunity for farmers to interact with community members, taking turns eating from one another's cornfields, sharing stories, and food preparation. In a way, it allows them to see beyond their small farms and become part of a more extensive cultural network representing an integrated life form with everything necessary for sustenance and well-being.

Native Americans are primarily known for their hunting and fishing skills, but they also have a vast knowledge of wild foods that can be harvested.

When my dad was growing up on a farm, he'd go out in the evening to cut hay with his mule and plow the fields with his horses. At some point during his working day, he came across an area with an enormous cattail patch.

The cattails were stacked to the field's sides, and their flat crowns hung low over the area. It wasn't until my father was older that he was told what the field was for, to hunt rabbits. The old-timers would lay water in the cattail field and wait for the rabbits to come to drink it. They'd then stand with their gun and shoot the rabbits as they gathered at the water.

This method, known as cattail lying, is used by various tribes today, although some variations exist on how it is executed.

It's easy to see why people used to do this, as my dad had a few rabbits now and then during his childhood. He didn't get into the actual hunting until years later, but he always has fond memories of those times with his mule.

I suspect this water method was so popular among tribes for a long time because of how much water they could obtain and how simple it was.

NATIVE AMERICANS WIDELY USED MEDICINAL PLANTS

Blackberries

The Cherokee used this fruit to ease a troubled stomach. They used blackberry to cure diarrhea and soothe sore tissues and joints (tea). Blackberry root can create an all-natural cough remedy with honey or maple syrup to treat sore throats. They have used the leaves to suck (bleeding) to soothe gum infections. Sometimes, to strengthen the whole immune system, this plant is perfect.

Sumac

This plant may be used in various herbal remedies, but this is one of the few plants employed to remedy eye problems by healers. Sumac decoctions were common as a gargle for sore throats and diarrhea treatment. The leaves and berries were blended into tea or made into a potion to soothe poison ivy to alleviate fever.

Mint

The Cherokee used to prepare mint tea to soothe digestion symptoms and help an irritated stomach; they also made a salve from its leaves to treat sore skin and rashes.

Rosemary

Native American tribes found this herb to be sacred. It was primarily used as an analgesic to relieve muscle pain. This herb improves concentration, relieves muscle pain and spasms, and stimulates the circulatory and nervous systems. Therefore, the immune reaction is reinforced, and indigestion is treated.

The Bark of Black Gum

The Cherokee also used to produce light tea from twigs and black gum bark to ease chest pains.

Red Clover

Healers have also used this herb to cure asthma and respiratory issues. In addition, new studies have shown that red clover helps prevent heart risk by increasing breathing and reducing cholesterol.

Greenbriar

This root tea has been used to purify blood or relieve joint pain. In addition, a salve combined with hog lard from leaves and bark was prepared by some healers, which was applied to mild sores, scalds, and burns.

Cattail

This is one of the most common medicinal plants used by indigenous people for food and also as defensive medicine. It helps to recover from illness, as it is a food that is easily digestible. Because it can be used in numerous dishes, it is named the swamp supermarket.

Sage

Sage is commonly used as a seasoning, but it was a sacred plant for many indigenous populations as it was thought to purify solid energies and cleanse the body of toxic energy. In addition, it has been used as a remedy to tackle medical conditions such as abdominal cramps, spasms, fractures, wounds, colds, and influenza.

Hummingbird Blossom

The American Indians used this herb, also known as the buck brush, to treat mouth and throat issues, cysts, fibroid tumors, and inflammation. It may be a potion to help treat wounds, sores, and injuries.

A diuretic that increases kidney function may be developed using the roots of such herb. The early colonists used this unusual plant as a substitute for black tea. The new studies have also shown that the buck brush helps control the lymph stream's elevated blood pressure and blockages.

Slippery Elm

The Native Americans made bowstrings, yarn, fabric, and rope using the inner bark. Tea was prepared to soothe toothaches, nasal irritations, skin issues, intestinal pain, sore throats, and even leaf and bark were used against spider bites.

Rose of the Wild

This herb was used as a preventive and a remedy for mild common cold by Native Americans. In addition, the tea is a stimulant and a mild diuretic for the bladder and kidneys. For a sore throat, a petal injection was used.

Ginger of the Wild

Healers use this herb to treat earaches and ear infections. They also found that a gentle tea for the rootstock stimulates the digestive system, reduces bloating, and aids in bronchialdiseases and exhaustion.

Lavender

Healers have used this herb as a medication for fatigue, anxiety, tension, headaches, and exhaustion. Antiseptic and anti-inflammatory properties are found in the essential oil. Insect bites and burns can be soothed with infusions.

Honeysuckle

Native Americans used this herb to cure asthma, but it has medical applications for hepatitis, rheumatoid arthritis, and mumps. It also helps in upper respiratory tract infections, such as pneumonia.

Cactus of the Prickly Pear

This plant is used both as a diet and as a medicine. Native Americans produced a poultice from developed sheets as an antiseptic for treating burns, boils, and wounds. Tea was prepared to treat urine infections and to improve the immune system. The study further shows that cholesterol can be decreased, and even heart failure and diet-related diabetes can be avoided.

Mullein

It was a tobacco-like plant and was mainly used to treat respiratory disorders. To relieve swelling in the joints, paws, or feet, Native Americans created mixtures from the roots.

Ashwagandha

This plant was important for healers because of its various unusual medicinal uses. It treats bone weakness, muscle wasting, stiffness, loss of teeth, and memory loss, as well as rheumatism. And it can be used as a sedative. It also has an ultimate rejuvenating effect on the body as it improves stamina. Using the leaves and root bark as an antibiotic is often essential. When made into a poultice, it helps reduce swelling and controls pain. Caution is advised when using this plant, as it is toxic.

Uva Ursi

It is also known as Bearberry and Bear grape due to the bear's affection for this plant's fruits. Native Americans used this herb mainly to treat bladder and urinary tract diseases.

Devil's Claw

American Indians used it to treat various ailments, from fever to benign skin conditions, and to improve metabolism and arthritis, even though the name suggests it is a toxic plant. While a decoction made from the plant's roots prevents stiffness and helps with sores, joint diseases, gout, back pain, headache, and arthritis, the effects of diabetes can be reduced by the tea. Although medical treatment is not accessible, knowledge about herbs like this is the only doctorthat will save you.

Origin of Licorice

This root is commonly used for flavoring candies, foods, and beverages. But

healers have also used it to treat stomach disorders, bronchitis, food poisoning, and chronic fatigue.

Salix (Willow)

Both the Greeks and American Indians valued willow bark for pain relief, and among the first therapeutic substances collected from the plants in 1852 was the herb's active ingredient, salicin. It proved to be a successful analgesic, yet it weakened the stomach. So the research was promoted to form a drug now manufactured as aspirin, which is identical and safer.

Rosy Periwinkle (Catharanthus Roseus)

Both parts of the plant are venomous. In Rosy periwinkle, there are many compounds of therapeutic potential, two of which, vincristine and vinblastine, are essential drugs in treating leukemia and certain other cancers.

Yew (Taxus Baccata)

Native Americans used the Pacific yew from North America (Northwest) to treat skin cancer. A clinical study has shown that Taxol, a drug that has become an effective treatment for breast, ovarian and cervical cancer, is included in this plant. Fortunately, it was discovered that English yews have a particular compound in their leaves that can be converted into Taxol. Pharmaceutical companies are collecting yew hedge clippings for this purpose.

Chamomile (The Flower)

In the United States, chamomile is widely used for anxiety and relaxation as an anxiolytic and sedative, considered by few to be a cure-all. It is used in Europe for wound healing and minimizing swelling and inflammation. Few trials have investigated how well it operates for any disease. Chamomile is used as a compress and as for tea. It is considered safe by the FDA. Sleepiness triggered by drugs or other herbs or supplements can increase. Chamomile may interfere with how the body uses other medications, allowing the number of drugs to be too big in certain persons. Speak, as for any medicinal plant, with the healthcare provider before taking it.

Garlic (Root Cloves)

Garlic is used for cholesterol levels and control of blood pressure. It has antimicrobial effects. Reports from minor, short-term, and poorly defined trials suggest slight decreases may be induced by total and LDL cholesterol. The German research results on garlic's cholesterol-lowering influence have been distorted; however, with a positive impact, the FDA says. Researchers are currently studying the possible role of garlic in cancer prevention. The FDA considers garlic to be safe. It should not be mixed with warfarin since large amounts of garlic can induce clotting. Big doses must not be administered until oral surgery or surgical intervention for the same reason.

Feverfew (The Leaf)

Historically, Feverfew has been used as a cure for fever. It is still commonly used to treat arthritis and alleviate migraines. Any evidence has indicated that migraines can be avoided with any feverfew treatment. Among the adverse effects are oral ulcers and abdominal pain. People who suddenly avoid taking feverfew for migraines can have their headaches returned. It cannot be used with nonsteroidal anti-inflammatory drugs since they can impact how well feverfew performs. It cannot be used in combination with warfarin and other anticoagulant medications.

Ginger (The Root)

Ginger is used to minimizing pain and dizziness. The study indicates that ginger may decrease pain caused by pregnancy and chemotherapy. Surgery and motion-induced nausea are implicated in these areas under evaluation. Some side effects are gas, bloating, heartburn, and nausea.

Goldenseal (Rhizome, Racine)

Goldenseal is used to treat diarrhea, itchy eyes, and skin. It is used in the context of an antiseptic. It is also an unproven treatment for colds. Goldenseal contains berberine, a plant alkaloid with a long history of medicinal use in Ayurvedic and Chinese medicine. The efficacy of goldenseal for diarrhea has been proven through research. But it is not allowed because it could be unsafe in large quantities. It can relieve skin, mouth, stomach, and gastric pain. It is not recommended due to the endangered species status of the plant.

Ginseng (The Root)

As a tonic and aphrodisiac, ginseng is also used as a cure-all. The analysis remains uncertain regarding how well it does, mainly owing to the difficulty in defining "vitality" and "quality of life." The accuracy of sold ginseng varies greatly. Side effects of its use include elevated blood pressure and tachycardia.

Milk Thistle (The Fruit)

Milk thistle treats liver problems and high cholesterol and reduces cancer cell formation. It is native to the Mediterranean area. For thousands of years, it has been used for different diseases, including liver problems. Although the conclusions of the analysis are unclear, there are some positive details.

Valeriana (The Root)

Valerian is used for sleeplessness management and anxiety relief. The studies indicate valerian can be a beneficial sleep aid, but no well-designed research has supported the claims. Valerian is used in the United States as a flavoring for root beer and other foods. Chat with the medical professional before taking it, as with any herbal plant.

Saint John's Wort (Flower, Leaf)

Saint John's Wort is regarded as an antidepressant. The latest findings have not established that depression has more than a negligible impact. Further research is required to decide the best dosage. The sensitivity to light is a side effect, although this is mainly noted in patients taking heavy doses of the drug. St. John's wort may induce harmful interaction with other widely used drugs. Before consuming this plant, please consult with a healthcare provider.

PATHOLOGIES TREATABLE USING NATIVE AMERICAN HERBS

Diarrhea

Diarrhea is often triggered by mild outbreaks of diet-borne diseases or food poisoning. Often, certain infections can cause moderate diarrhea.

Eating so much food, such as new fruit, consuming foods that you are resistant to or intolerant of, such as milk products, or developing digestive problems, such as colitis and irritable bowel syndrome, are other sources of diarrhea.

When the large intestine and colon require food waste to travel rapidly, it does not hold moisture and nutrients. The colon will also draw water from the body and eliminate extra feces in a rush. Without vital nutrients, the body will get dehydrated.

Astringent Herbs

The intestinal mucous membranes are helped by astringent herbs such as blackberry leaf or raspberry leaf to "dry up" per cup, using one heaping teaspoon. Drink about half a cup each hour. There is some debate about using these teas whilebreastfeeding.

Carob powder can be broken into a fiber-rich (electrolyte

hydrating) industrial replenishing beverage. Do not give carob to children unless directed by a physician.

In cranberry extract, the astringent characteristic is also present (Vaccinium myrtillus). Therefore, do not use blackberry if taking anticoagulants (blood thinners). Theoretically, it is even possible to link bilberry with diabetes medications.

Agrimony is a popular treatment for diarrhea. However, it may have an anticoagulant effect and may increase blood pressure. If you are concerned about these health issues, talk to your health care provider before you start taking this herb.

Inflammation Reducers

A fruit-dependent flavonoid, quercetin, may help reduce inflammation.

Chamomile (Matricaria recutita) is often taken as a tea. However, chamomile may interact with hormonal therapies that can cause symptoms in people allergic to ragweed.

Althea officinalis (marshmallow root) should be taken in the form of cold water. Simply soak some of the seeds in a liter of pressurized water overnight. Consume the mixture throughout the day. Marshmallows may interact with some medications, such as lithium, administered orally. Ulmus fulva or Althaea Officinalis (slippery elm powder) may soothe the bowels (marshmallow root powder). Make a paste with the powder and a smaller volume of water. Pour most of the water steadily and then simmer until it reaches one pint. Slippery elm has a well-known reputation for interacting incorrectly with some medicines.

How to Calm the Fever

This natural treatment will help you stay calm and comfortable when coping with a low temperature.

If your forehead feels feverish, you should search for acetaminophen (Tylenol) or ibuprofen (Advil) to decrease the temperature.

But don't be scared to let it run its course whether the fever is 101 °F (38.3 ° C) or lower. However, if you're uncomfortable and want to take steps, consider some home-cure remedies to help tame the flames.

How to calm the fever? Soak yourself in a lukewarm bath. If you have a headache, this temperature will sound good enough, and the tub can help lower the body temperature. You don't want to put down a fever immediately; the treatment sends blood rush to tissues (internal), which is how the body protects itself against cold. Instead of cooling down, the interior warms up.

A sponge bath is a good choice. Sponging high-heat areas with cold water such as the armpits and groin will help decrease the temperature as water evaporation begins.

Place cool and damp washcloths on the forehead and back of the neck.

Drink a little tea. Brew the yarrow tea in a cup. This herb expands the lungs and causes the process of sweating, which brings fever to an end. Steep a tablespoon of the herb for 10 minutes in a cup of freshly distilled water. Just let it cool. Before you begin sweating, drink one or two cups.

Another vine, the elderflower, also improves sweating. And it appears to be helpful for some complications related to flu and colds, such as excessive mucus production. Mix two teaspoons, create the herb infusion in a cup of boiling water, and let it steep for 15 minutes. Strain the elderflower. Drink for the duration of the fever three times a day. Elderberries are also rich in antioxidants that boost immunity.

Drink a cup of hot tea with ginger, which often triggers transpiration. To create the tea, brew a half teaspoon of minced ginger root in a cup of boiled water, then strain. Drink afterward.

Willow bark can help ease a headache and is a good aspirin alternative. Consume it in a powdered form, as a tincture, or even as a tea.

Get it spicy. Sprinkle cayenne pepper on the diet while you have a fever. Capsaicin, the alarmingly hot compound used in hot peppers, is one of the key ingredients. Cayenne helps you sweat and promotes fast blood flow as well.

Indigested Causes
Dyspepsia, Indigestion

Indigestion is also caused by overeating, chewing too hard, or consuming too much greasy or hot food. It can also be caused by psychological conditions, including depression or anxiety.

Indigestion can be more frequent in individuals with the following disorders:

- Ulcer's peptics

- Pancreatitis
- Breast problems
- Anomaly in the bile ducts or pancreas
- Gallstones
- Gastritis

Natural Treatments

While there is little literature on natural indigestion cures, peppermint tea or consuming ginger can be prescribed by alternative medicine practitioners to ease the digestive tract after a meal.

Studies indicate that other specific herbal therapies can provide indigestion relief as well.

Extract the Artichoke Leaf

Artichoke is rich in antioxidants and antimicrobial properties and is popular in Mediterranean countries. It has been used to prevent liver injury, decrease cholesterol levels, and manage dyspepsia.

A 2015 study tracked men and women aged 17 to 80 who suffered from stomach discomfort or vomiting in the case of nausea or bloating over three months. Since drinking a supplementary blend of artichoke leaf extract and ginger for around two weeks, only the group who consumed the blend felt reduced symptoms. Researchers noticed at four weeks that the medication minimized indigestion in more than 60% of cases. They theorized that the antispasmodic effects of artichoke leaf extract and its capacity to facilitate bile acid secretion also assist gastrointestinal transit, helping to relieve bloating and fullness.

Remedies Using Herbs

It is too early to prescribe some natural medications to solve indigestion because adequate studies have not been performed. Therefore, it is necessary to remember that self-management of the disease, abandonment, or discontinuation of routine care can have vital implications. Contact your health care provider if you consider using herbal medications in indigestion care.

Slowing down while you eat can help to decrease the risk of indigestion. These preventive methods involve minimizing caffeine consumption and carbonated beverages, using calming approaches such as deep relaxation and meditation instead of two to three bigger meals, and preparing fewer, more frequent meals.

HOW TO CULTIVATE AND PREPARE HERBS

The cultivation technique of the Native Americans is a resource for understanding some of the most practical approaches for living passed down from generation to generation. It contains tips on growing plants, fishing, hunting deer or foxes, finding shelter in various terrains, and more. The report also has information on creating fire by using natural elements found in nature, such as rubbing sticks together or using flint and steel. Unfortunately, the strategies shared are often forgotten or not spoken about as much in modern society with all its complexities.

Proponents of these techniques include medicine men, shamans, older women, spiritual leaders, and grandmothers from many Native American cultures across North America. They use these techniques within their traditional practices and benefit family, friends, and communities. The commonalities among these groups are the people's desire to better themselves each day, with a healthy mind/body connection. They recognize that giving back to the earth is a way of giving back to their creator ancestors. These Native American Cultivation Techniques are used in daily ceremonies for prayer, healing, and community building.

Soil Preparation

I firmly believe that the soil where you plant your seeds is one of gardening's most essential aspects. The soil must be well aerated, have a high nutrient content, and be sufficiently acidic for healthy plants. Planting directly into the ground grown in highly acidic chemical fertilizer won't yield the best results! Luckily all of these points are here in great detail, so I'll tell you what it is said:

"How to choose a healthy seedbed: Plant too deeply, and your plant will be unable to reach vital root cells on which it depends for nourishment; plant more shallowly, and you risk having roots wandering around indiscriminately. Directly dig into the soil, avoiding rocks and any hard, woody material, or scratching the surface with a hand cultivator or rake to make it more brittle. The key is to avoid compacting and deepening the topsoil. How not to choose a seedbed: Never plant into a cradle that has been fertilized with manure. You may grow beautiful carrot tops while the roots are rotting away."

How to loosen up heavy soil: Dig in plenty of organic matter such as compost, rotted manure, well-rotted farm animal bedding, or peat moss. Also, use organic matter such as seaweed, alfalfa meal, or perlite (small chips of volcanic glass that expand to a thickness of about 1/8 inch, an organic "grow-stone" that helps retain moisture). How not to loosen up heavy soil: Compacted soil needs more water and work out much more slowly. Try using a slow-release fertilizer (asopposed to "instant").

Plant Selection

Variety is essential in making your garden wildlife-friendly, as it breaks up what might otherwise be monotonous surroundings and provides a more exciting view.

Choosing "naturally diverse" plants will help your garden to remain healthy and productive. Look for plants adapted to specific locations and selected based on their ability to thrive in your area. You could even choose a few species of trees or shrubs that suit the climate for which you have decided to plant a small stand.

How to Collect Natural Fertilizer

Some of the best sources of organic matter include pine needles, grass clippings, and leaves. Be careful not to pile up dead leaves; a very heavy application (or too much of one kind) will make the soil too acidic.

When it comes to the amount of leaf mold you should add to your compost pile or the amount of fertilizer you should add to your soil, make sure you don't overdo it.

An easy way to produce leaf mulch is by cutting grass with a lawnmower. You can usually get rid of unwanted vegetation (such as dandelions) this way as well. Then, after you have missed the grass, mow it again so that it looks like what might be called "grass clippings."

One of the best natural fertilizers is chicken manure. You can obtain it by allowing sources of chicken waste to build up in any coop. Old newspapers placed in the enclosure will help capture this waste and minimize odor.

Grow Your Food All Year Long

If you live anywhere in Minnesota—or any other challenging winter climate—chances, are you can grow food all winter long! Because it's cold outside, Native Americans didn't spend much time on their crops for the same reasons many people today don't grow their food. They have their hunting and gathering spots that they know well enough to invest much time in them. They are also aware that there will be times when there is little food for them due to drought or other factors beyond their control. So, they find times when they can produce a surplus of food and store it for consumption when it is scarce.

Harvest season is a time of year that everyone looks forward to.

The Native Americans are skilled at preserving food. There are tips on keeping greens, roots, and fruits used in recipes later in the year. You can check some of their methods.

If you are unfamiliar with plants, you need to find out what is edible so that you do not risk your health or your life while trying to survive. Mistakes while foraging for food can kill you, and all the time spent on education may be misspent if you do not know how to identify the most basic vegetation types.

Native Americans living in forested areas know how to navigate them with an eye out for edible plants. Unfortunately, these wild foods are often overlooked by others interested in hunting games or growing their food. However, that doesn't mean it's not growing season for some vegetables.

Essential Tools

Because when herbal plants are being prepared, they come in various ways, different tools are essential depending on what preparation is at hand. However, the following list of basic tools is mainly needed for house-made preparations.

- Scissors and baskets: In harvesting herbal plants, a basket is essential for collecting. It is the carrier of the gathered plants. As for the scissors, it is needed for the picking part. Considering how thick stems could be, ahigh-quality pair of scissors is suggested.

- Fine mesh sieve (In all sizes): It is essential to have numerous sizes. They can be used when the preparation needs separating different mixtures or when a texture is required to be achieved. The largest one is the most helpful for tinctures or infusions.

- Potato ricer: It is suggested to be the cheaper alternative for the tincture press. It is another tool used to strain infused oils or tinctures. It is assured that it will be used until the last extract.

- Mortar and pestle: They are used to grind different herbs. From the manual grinding, an extract will be gathered from the plants.

- Spice grinder: More than its grinding feature, it could also store different herbs, and all will be preserved with its medicinal quality and properties. Herbals are known to quickly lose their quality, making this tool very helpful to have in store.

- Kitchen scale: For various recipes of preparation, precise and accurate weights of ingredients are needed. This is why the scale is included in the list of most essential tools. Likewise, for herbal tinctures and teas, precision and accuracy are crucial.

- Stainless steel funnel: This is used in storing and moving herbal medicines from different jars or plastics.

- Tea press: A tea press is the most helpful way to make

large batches of teas. It can be used for infusions too. In addition, the tea press could contribute to taking herbal plant extracts.

- Tea strainer: This tool ensures that no residuals are present in every tea drink. Moreover, they are also reported to keep volatile aromatic oils in every sip.
- Electric teapot: It is the easiest way to have hot water, an essential element in various preparations. It is dominantly present in each practice.

These tools are commonly seen at home, as this book recommends home- friendly procedures. However, people are persuaded to be more resourceful and creative. If these tools are kept aside, the preparation of herbs will also be cheaper.

PREPARING HERBAL REMEDIES

In many countries, herbal remedies are still widespread—often the only treatment available. However, they are also becoming more mainstream in North America and Europe.

Herbal remedies such as infusions, decoctions, syrups, compresses, poultices, and ointments can treat many common ailments. Each of these is prepared in a certain wayand is appropriate for only certain herbs.

Recipes will always vary, depending on the herbs used and the symptoms being treated. For this reason, no specific individual recipes are included, simply a general preparation description of how to prepare them.

If you're new to using and making herbal remedies, consult a qualified, reputable herbalist or a health professional for detailed information on properties and preparations. Herbal treatments can be dangerous if you don't know the properties of the herb and its consequences.

Infusions

Infusions are the most straightforward remedy to prepare at home. An infusion is a tea and can be brewed from either dried or fresh herbs.

A herb's water-soluble components are extracted via infusions. The hot water releases volatile oils (also known as essential oils) within the plant. The oils are usually the ones that provide the most health benefits. Plant parts that grow above the ground, such as leaves, flowers, and stems, are used to make infusions.

Use two tablespoons of dried herbs or half a cup of freshly washed herbs (leaves or flowers) for every two cups of boiling water. Use a ceramic or glass pot and fresh filtered water. Pour boiling water over fresh or dried herbs and allow them to brew for up to 15 minutes. Strain and your infusionwill be ready to use.

Drink infusions, either hot or cold, up to four times daily. Infusions will keep for about a week in the refrigerator. After that, you can add lemon juice or honey as a sweetener.

You can also inhale the vapors, depending on which herb you use and what symptoms you relieve. Use infusions externally to form a poultice applied to the skin, as a rinse for hair, or added to bathwater as a skin soother.

Decoctions

Decoctions are prepared from combinations of dried or fresh herbs, fresh bark, dried roots, or stems simmered in pure filtered water. Use two tablespoons of dried herbs or one to two cups of bark, roots, or stems for every two cups of water.

Place the ingredients into boiling water (use a non-reactive enamel pan) and let it simmer gently for 30 minutes. Strain out the herbal product before you use a decoction. Like teas, these will keep refrigerated for up to a week.

When ingested, decoctions can have substantial effects, including dizziness and nausea, so use them carefully. Also, dilute to prepare as a drink since they are much more potent than infusions.

They make excellent compresses, applied externally to bruises, sprains, and strained muscles.

Decoctions are one of the primary therapies in Traditional Chinese Medicine. Many formulas have been created to treatvarious conditions; some are still in use today.

Herbal Syrups

Syrups are made similarly to decoctions, using herbs and water. Boil the mix of herbs and water gently until the liquid reduces by half. Strain out the spices, add one to two tablespoons of unpasteurized organic honey for every two cups of liquid, and store the syrup in the refrigerator.

A simple thyme cough syrup can be made using 1/4 cup dried or 1/2 cup fresh thyme leaves in one and a quarter cups of water. Simmer the thyme and water for 20 minutes, or until the water is reduced to half. Remove from the heat and strain the thyme through cheesecloth, squeezing it to get as much liquid as possible. Add the juice of half a lemon and two tablespoons of unpasteurized, unfiltered honey.

Other herbs that work well for making syrups to fight colds and flu are sage, ginger, horehound, and peppermint.

Tinctures

A tincture is made with plant parts—flowers, leaves, or

roots—steeped in alcohol. Since alcohol is more effective than water in extracting the herb's active constituents, smaller herbs are required. Tinctures are very concentrated extracts, so they are incredibly effective. They keep for a long time; they are one of the best ways to use your herbs. Because this is a cold preparation method, the volatile ingredients are not lost as they can be with infusions, teas, or decoctions, all of which require heat.

Use a sealable glass jar to make your tincture. Pack the pot full of freshly washed and dry herbs or a quarter full of dried herbs.

Fill the jar with quality vodka. This is one of the purest food-grade alcohols because it is flavorless, colorless, and odorless. Use only alcohol that's 80 proof or higher. Stir with a plastic knife or spoon to release any trapped air bubbles.

Seal the jar with a layer of wax paper and screw on the lid tightly. Set the pot away for up to a month in a cold, dark location, shaking it once or twice a day.

At the end of that time, filter the contents through cheesecloth layers or a coffee filter. Finally, seal the resulting tincture in a sterile dark-colored jar or bottle.

Label your tincture with ingredients, date, and the recommended dosage and use. Because of the preservation action of the alcohol, tinctures may last up to 5 years.

Compresses

Compresses are cloths soaked in a liquid and applied externally to an aching muscle or a bruised and swollen area.

Use a tincture or a decoction of a herb recommended for the specific ailment to help treat aches, sore throats, and skin conditions.

Compresses can be used either cold or hot. Hot compresses ease muscle pain, while cold compresses relieve headaches and reduce swelling. Begin by making a strong tea or tincture. Take a small towel, a washcloth, or a piece of clean, dry gauze, depending on which part of your body, and dip it into the tea. Apply it to the affected area. Once it cools, re- soak it in the warmed tea and reapply as often as needed.

Herbal Poultices

Poultices help draw out infections, treat boils, relieve inflammation, and draw out poisons from insect bites. Use them to ease chest congestion.

Begin by mashing or mincing the chosen herb into a pulp. Next, pour boiling water over to cover and make a paste. Finally, use a mortar, pestle, or even a food processor or blender. Try olive or almond oil in place of water.

Allow it to cool, and then spread it directly on the area you want to treat. Cover it with gauze or a bandage for as long as necessary.

Herbal Plasters

Plasters are like poultices, but there is one big difference. They aren't applied to the skin directly. Because they don't contact the skin, you can use spicier or hotter herbs with more excellent antiseptic and healing abilities. Ginger and mustard are often utilized for plasters.

The plant materials are often dried or powdered with plasters and mixed with a carrier like oatmeal, ground flax, or honey to make a paste when mixed with hot water.

The resulting paste is spread onto a cloth, set in place, and bound to the area with a strip of fabric. Test to ensure the plaster is not too hot before applying it. Allow up to four hours for the plaster to set.

Herbal Ointments

Is it an ointment, a salve, or a balm? These can all be described under the heading of ointments, but there are slight differences between them, mainly in their consistency and designated use. All are mixtures of herbal-infused oils and essential oils designed for external use. Wax helps form a protective layer on the skin and stiffness of the body during the preparation.

Balms are stiffest since many are used in twist-up dispensers—think of lip balm or deodorants. There is a higher ratio of wax to oil in balms, and usually, the essential oil is added for its more robust aroma and healing properties.

Salves are mainly made with herbal-infused oils and beeswax and do not usually contain essential oils. As a result, they are softer than balms and easily spread over a bruise or injury.

Ointments are almost identical to salves, with an oilier texture and essential oil content for healing. Due to the higher oil content, the skin easily absorbs the healing components. Vegetable oils are the best choice, specifically coconut oil. Other choices are olive oil, almond oil, or avocado oil. Choose an organic oil.

Begin making a salve by creating an oil infusion. Place your chosen herbs and oil in a glass or enamel pot over a larger pot with water—an improvised double boiler. Bring the water to a boil. Reduce to a simmer and allow the oil andherbs to infuse for up to an hour.

Remove the infused oil from heat and strain it through cheesecloth layers, squeezing as much oil from the herbs as possible. Measure, so you know how much wax is required. You require an ounce of beeswax for each cup of oil.

Place the wax in a clean pot over low heat, pour in the infused oil, and allow them to combine as the wax melts. Pour the resulting mixture into sterile jars and cover.

TRADITIONAL REMEDIES FORCOMMON AILMENTS

Allergies

Mucus production, itchy eyes, and a runny nose are common symptoms of allergies. The remedies here can help, but you can also help by changing your diet during allergy season. For example, milk and other dairy items can promote mucus production; therefore, cut them out of your diet to aid healing.

The herbs used for allergies are nettle, elderflower, and echinacea. For asthma, the herbs used are nettle, chamomile, and echinacea.

General Asthma Remedies

Make an infusion of nettle and take 400–600 ml daily for no more than three months at a time. To prepare a pot of the infusion, use 20 g dried or 30 g fresh herbs. Add them to a warmed teapot. Pour 500 ml of boiling water into the pot. Infuse for 10 minutes, then pour some out into a cup, but don't exceed the dosage measurements. Sugar or honey can be used if desired. The surplus infusion can be kept in the fridge for up to 24 hours.

The second general remedy is to make an infusion of nettle and elderflower. To prepare this infusion, use one teaspoon dried or two teaspoons of each fresh herb to 300 ml of water. This is one dose. Make the infusion like tea, with the herbs in a strainer and boiling water poured over. Cover with a lid and infuse for 5–10 minutes before removing the herbs and strainer. Again, feel free to add sweetener or honey if desired.

Hay Fever

Make an infusion of elderflower and take 300–450 ml a day. Drink the infusion daily for a few months before and during allergy season. To prepare a pot of the infusion, use 20 g of dried or 30 g of fresh herbs. Add them to a warmed teapot. Pour 500 ml boiling water into the pot. Infuse for 10 minutes, then follow the dosage measurements. Feel free to add sweeteners or honey if you need it. You can store the extra infusion in the fridge for up to 24 hours.

Wheezing

Make an infusion of two herbs: thyme and nettle. To prepare an infusion pot, use 15 g of each herb. Add them to a warmed teapot. Pour 710 ml of boiling water into the pot. Infuse for 10 minutes. Drink it throughout the day. Feel free to add sweeteners or honey if needed.

The second remedy is to make an infusion with German chamomile.

To prepare the infusion, use two heaping teaspoons of chamomile to 150 ml of water. This is one dose. Make the infusion like tea, with the herbs in a strainer and boiling water poured over. Cover with a lid and infuse for 10 minutes. Inhale the steam before removing the herbs and strainer. Drink the infusion, and feel free to add sweetener or honey if necessary.

Asthma or Infections

This remedy has a couple of different options. First, you can take capsules or a tincture of echinacea. To make the capsule, fill a capsule case with about 500 mg of powdered echinacea. Take one capsule three times a day. Alternatively, sprinkle the same amount of powder on food or in water. For the tincture, take ½ teaspoon 1:5 tincture with water 2–3 times a day.

EAR, NOSE, AND THROAT

Bronchitis/Chest Cold

Eucalyptus leaves are an excellent remedy for getting rid of mucus. It is also a good antiseptic and helps with many respiratory ailments. In addition, Elecampane is a root used to help with most chest infections and complaints.

Elecampane should not be taken if you are breastfeeding or pregnant. You should also not give eucalyptus to children or infants.

The first remedy is an infusion of thyme. You can have up to 750 ml daily; however, a good option is to have 100 ml three times a day. Use 20 g of dried or 30 g of fresh herbs to make an infusion pot. Please place them in a teapot that has been warmed. Fill the saucepan halfway with boiling water. Allow for a 10-minute infusion before pouring some into a cup, but don't exceed the suggested dosage. You can sweetenthe infusion if you want.

For coughs and bronchitis, you can make a decoction of elecampane. You can add 5 g of eucalyptus leaf for acute coughs and bronchitis and 5 g of licorice powder for flavor. Drink about 300 ml of the decoction each day. Place 20 g of elecampane root (or 15 g elecampane and 5 g eucalyptus for acute coughs) and 750 ml of water in a saucepan to make a decoction. Bring to a boil, then reduce to low heat for 20-30 minutes. It should be reduced until just 500 ml of liquid is left. Sieve the mixture, reserving the liquid but tossing out the herbs. Refrigerate any leftover decoction for up to 48 hours.

Remember, don't take this remedy if you are pregnant.

For an external chest rub (never taken internally), mix five drops of thyme essential oil, five drops of eucalyptus essential oil, and two teaspoons of olive oil. Use up to twice a day on your chest and back. Never ingest this mixture, and don't use it if you are pregnant.

Fever

You can make an infusion of yarrow and elderberry; however, this remedy shouldn't be taken if you are pregnant. To prepare the infusion, use ½ teaspoon of yarrow and ½ teaspoon of elderberry to 100 ml of water. This is one dose. Make the infusion like tea, with the herbs in a strainer and boiling water poured over. Before removing the herbs and strainer, cover with a lid and steep for 10 minutes. If necessary, sweeten with honey or a sweetener. You may consume up to 600 ml of water each day.

You can take a whole onion and bake it at 400°F for 40 minutes as an alternative remedy. Mix honey with an equal amount of onion juice. You can take one or two teaspoons of the remedy every hour, but don't exceed eight times a day. You can also reduce a fever without herbal help by bathing in cool water.

You can make an infusion of yarrow, boneset, and cayenne for high fever. Boneset is a new herb for this book. You will use the aerial parts of the plant for this remedy. You should not use this remedy if you are pregnant. To prepare the infusion, use one teaspoon of dried boneset, one teaspoon of dried yarrow, and a pinch of cayenne to 150 ml of water. This is one dose. Make the infusion like tea, with the herbs in a strainer and boiling water poured over. Cover with a lid and infuse for five minutes before removing the herbs and strainer. Feel free to add a sweetener, honey, ginger, or cinnamon for flavor if you need to.

You can take up to 600 ml of the infusion a day.

Stuffy Nose and Sinus Infections

For congestion issues, the remedy is to inhale the steam of infusions or essential oils.

The first remedy is inhaling the steam of an infusion. To prepare the infusion, use 15 g of dried herbs to 750 ml of water. Make the infusion like tea by straining the herbs and pouring boiling water over them. Before removing the herbs and filter, cover with a lid and steep for 5-10 minutes. Theninhale the steam for 10 minutes.

You can also use German chamomile, following the exact directions above. You can also exchange the herbs with 5-10 drops of eucalyptus essential oil or chamomile essential oil and follow the rest of the suggestions above.

Sore Throat and Laryngitis

All these remedies will help sore throats and can also be beneficial to healing laryngitis. You can also simply gargle with warm water and salt for laryngitis.

For a sore throat, you can gargle 20 ml of lemon juice. If it's too strong for you, you can dilute it with some water and honey. Alternatively, gargle with five teaspoons of lemon juice with a pinch of powdered cayenne pepper.

Another remedy is to create an infusion of sage. Do not take this remedy if you are pregnant. To prepare the infusion, use one teaspoon of dried or two teaspoons of fresh herb to 250 ml of water. This is one dose. Make the infusion like tea, with the herbs in a strainer and boiling water poured over. Before removing the herbs and strainer, cover with a lid and steep for 10 minutes. Allow it to cool somewhat, so it doesn't burn your mouth, then gargle and swallow the infusion. To increase its effectiveness, add 5 ml of vinegar and honey.

Garlic, ginger, and lemon juice can also be used together. To make this juice, crush a clove of garlic. Wait 10 minutes before you use it. Then, mix the crushed garlic with a similar amount of grated fresh ginger, the juice from one lemon, and 150 ml of warm water. Drink up to 450 ml a day. This remedy is also effective for colds.

Gargling a decoction of echinacea root can also be an effective remedy. To create a decoction, combine 20 g of dried root and 750 ml of water in a pot.

Bring to a boil, then reduce to low heat for 20-30 minutes. It should be reduced until just 500 ml of liquid remains. Keep the liquid and discard the roots after sieving the mixture. Refrigerate any leftover decoction for up to 48 hours. Gargle 2½ tablespoons three times a day.

MEDICINAL REMEDIES FOR YOUR CHILDREN

2-12 Months

Geranium (Pelargonium graveolens)

This floral oil has been used to treat bruises, burns, congested skin, dermatitis, eczema, oily complexions, tonsillitis, sore throats, and nervous tension. However, it can cause dermatitis in susceptible skin.

Tangerine/Mandarin (Citrus reticulata)

This essential oil is labeled as one or the other in most natural health stores and online. Therefore, you should include the Latin name of the oil.

This oil is known to help with congested and oily skin, lightening scars, skin toner, intestinal problems, digestive problems, insomnia, nervous tension, and restlessness.

Eucalyptus (Eucalyptus globulus)

Well known for being used in vaporizers and other diffusion devices, eucalyptus has been used to open nasal passages and congested chests.

It can also help treat insect bites and skin infections and ease muscular aches and pains, sprains, and throat infections. It is also effective in treating bronchitis, sinusitis, colds, flu, and measles.

1-5 Years

Palmarosa (Cymnopogon martinii)

Acne, dermatitis, minor skin infections, scars, facials, oily skin, dry skin, and intestinal infections have all been relieved by this essential oil.

5-12 Years

Clary Sage (Salvia sclarea)

This is another strong essential oil, but it's suitable for this age range. I wouldn't make it the mainstay of a blend because it's a little more potent than before. However, for a tablespoon, two to three drops should be enough. This oil is good to help with acne, dandruff, oily skin and hair, muscular aches and pains, intestinal cramps, and flatulence.

Nutmeg (Myristica fragrans)

This aromatic oil is used to help treat muscular aches and pains, flatulence, indigestion, nausea, and bacterial infections.

REMEDIES FOR A RADIANT HEALTH

Acne

This happens when the sebaceous glands get infected and, as a result, shoot out painful bumps—what we all call "pimples." Acne affects all age groups and can appear on any body part.

Witch Hazel Toner

Ingredients:

- Three tablespoons of rosemary oil
- 1 cup witch hazel

Tools Needed:
- Colored glass bottle (dark)
- Cotton (cosmetic pad)

Instructions:

1. Put all ingredients into a dark-colored glass bottle and shake.
2. Prepare a cotton cloth, dip this in the mixture, and apply it on the surface affected every morning and evening until the acne disappears from your skin.

Sage–Chamomile Gel

Ingredients:

- Three teaspoons of powdered sage leaf
- 1 cup water
- Three teaspoons chamomile
- 1/8 cup aloe vera gel

Tools Needed:
- Saucepan Cheesecloth
- Glass jar Cotton

Instructions:

1. Put the saucepan on medium heat and add the sage leaf, chamomile, and water. Let it simmer, then remove from heat when it reduces by half.
2. Let it cool for 3 minutes.
3. Prepare a cheesecloth, use it to cover the edge of the funnel, and then pour all the mixture to the last drop into a bowl through the funnel.
4. Add the aloe vera gel to the mixture, and mix to blend.
5. Pour into the jar and store in a fridge.
6. Dip the cotton into the mixture and apply it to the affected skin every morning and evening.

Advice:

- Anyone allergic to any plant type in the same family as sage leaf and chamomile should avoid using this remedy.

Allergies

This abnormal effect of some substances causes the immune system to react badly. These substances are found in many products, including drinks, foods, and even the environment we live in.

Cattail Tincture

Ingredients:

- Four oz. 90% unflavored vodka
- Four oz. dried cattail

Tools Needed:
- Sterilized pint jar
- Cabinet Cheesecloth

Instructions:

1. Put the cattail in the sterilized pint jar and add the vodka. Make sure it slightly covers the top of the cattail.
2. Replace the jar cap, make sure it tightly covers the jar, and then shake gently to mix.
3. Store for about 8–12 weeks and shake to mix twice daily.
4. Dampen the cheesecloth at the mouth of the funnel, pour the tincture into another sterilized jar and drain till all the water comes out. Dispose of the herbs and sieve into a clean glass bottle (preferably dark-colored).
5. Take eight drops every day until the mixture finishes. If it's too firm, add some water or juice to dilute.

Advice:

- Do not use it if you're allergic to anything that falls under the same plant family as cattail.
- It's also not suitable for use by pregnant women and nursing mothers.

Garlic–Ginkgo Syrup

Ingredients:

- 3 oz. fresh or freeze-dried garlic, chopped
- 3 oz. Ginkgo Biloba, crushed or chopped
- 2 ½ cup water
- 2 cups of local honey

Tools Needed:
- One saucepan Measuring cups (glass)
- Sterilized jar

Instructions:

1. Put the garlic and Ginkgo Biloba in a saucepan with some water and boil on low heat. Cover it partially anddrain some water out of it.
2. Pour the contents of the saucepan into a glass measuring cup, then with a piece of cheesecloth on the mouth, drain back into the saucepan and wring till there is no water left.

Advice:

- If you're on antidepressants, you're strongly advised not to use this herbal remedy.

- Children under the age of ten should only take ½–1 teaspoon of this remedy three times per day.

Anxiety

Many herbal therapies have been tested to cure anxiety, but further study clarifies the hazards and benefits. This is what we know and do not know.

Kava

Kava proved to be a potential anxiety remedy. However, records of significant liver injury, also for short-term usage, prompted the FDA to provide recommendations on using kava-containing dietary supplements. Although these original liver toxicity findings have been disputed, have special care and include your specialist in the decision if you think about using kava items.

Passionflower

A few limited clinical trials indicate that the passionflower can assist with anxiety. Unfortunately, Passionflowers are mixed with other herbs in several consumer items, rendering it hard to discern each plant's distinctive characteristics. It is usually considered healthy when consumed as instructed, although some reports have shown it can induce drowsiness, dizziness, and confusion.

Valerian

Individuals that used valerian showed less distress and tension in several tests. However, people have reported no advantages in other studies. Valerian is usually considered healthy at prescribed levels. However, as long-term safety tests are incomplete unless the doctor approves, do not take this herb for more than a couple of weeks at a time. Any adverse effects, such as migraine, drowsiness, and dizziness, may be induced.

Lavender

Many types of research indicate that oral lavender or aromatherapy may decrease anxiety, although there is minimal and tentative research. Oral lavender can induce headaches and constipation. Appetite can also improve, the sedative impact of some drugs and supplements can improve, and low blood pressure can be induced.

Lemon Balm

Preliminary evidence suggests that certain signs of anxiety, including nervousness and excitability, may be minimized by a lemon balm. It is usually well-tolerated for short-term usage and is deemed healthy but may induce nausea and stomach pain.

The FDA is not regulating herbal products in the same way drugs do. However, the consistency of certain supplements can still be a concern, considering improved quality management legislation in force since 2010. Bear in mind: Natural does not necessarily mean safety.

Back Pain

Many herbal treatments can minimize drug consumption or offer additional value to current medical care to soothe your back.

Consume an Anti-Inflammatory Drink Every Day

As you consistently eat anti-inflammatory foods, several antioxidants, anti- inflammatory, and anti-cancer agents might build up in the blood. Over time, such potent agents can significantly decrease and prevent inflammatory reactions in the body.

It can help minimize your back pain to consume these nutritious beverages regularly.

Golden Milk

There are antioxidants, anti-arthritic, and anti-inflammatory effects of Turmeric, an Asian spice. Mixing a tiny amount (1/2 teaspoon) of turmeric powder in a cup of warm milk is a simple way to consume turmeric. You should add honey/stevia to the milk if you want a sweet flavor. Ideally, this drink before bedtime enables the anti-inflammatory mechanism to function when you are asleep.

In specific individuals, eating dairy products can raise inflammation. Trying plant-based milk, like almond milk, may be helpful.

Tart Cherry Juice

Cherries are high in antioxidants and anti-inflammatory

drugs. Cherry juice may help alleviate chronic or exercise-induced body pain. Cherry juice is widely accessible for purchase in food stores and includes tart cherry extract. Try to consume a cup of cherry juice normally and see whether it benefits back pain recovery.

Green Tea with Ginger

Ginger-green tea packets can be ordered from convenience stores, and you can comfortably enjoy a cup at work or at home. You can also try suffused herbal beverages, like ginger-green tea, which provides green tea and ginger's pain-relieving properties.

Such anti-inflammatory agents will build up in your body over time but having these beverages in your everyday diet can help decrease total inflammation and stop fresh inflammatory pain.

Bronchitis, Pneumonia, and Chest Cold

Allergies and infections mainly cause this condition. The area infected gets bloated and becomes painful, often leadingto constant coughing.

Rosemary–Licorice Root Vapor Treatment

Ingredients:

- 8 cups water
- 2 cups dried licorice root, chopped
- 1 cup fresh rosemary leaves, finely chopped

Tools Needed:
- Saucepan Bowl
- Big size bowl

Instructions:

1. Prepare a saucepan, pour some water, add the dried licorice root and boil over medium heat.
2. Then, let it simmer for 15 minutes.
3. After it simmers, pour it into a bowl and add the rosemary leaves.
4. Put the bowl on a small stool and get a big towel. Cover your head with this towel. Make sure your head faces the bowl directly.
5. Close your eyes during this procedure and inhale the steam from the mixture.
6. Do this again and again until you feel a significant improvement.

Advice:

- Not to be used by people having any of the following. High blood pressure, epilepsy, kidney-related issues, heart diseases, and diabetes.

Goldenseal Syrup

Ingredients:

- 1 oz. dried goldenseal root, chopped
- 2 oz. dried hyssop
- 2 ½ cups water
- 2 cups honey

Tools Needed:
- Saucepan
- Glass measuring cup
- Jar

Instructions:

1. Place a saucepan on low heat and add the goldenseal and water.
2. Leave on the heat until you notice the water has been reduced by half.
3. Pour the content of the saucepan into a glass cup and sieve through a dampened cheesecloth back into the saucepan.
4. Let it boil for about 2–5 minutes, add some honey, and stir until thoroughly mixed.

Advice:

- Not to be taken by pregnant women or nursing mothers.

- Not to be used by anyone who has epilepsy and high blood pressure
- It should not be administered to children under the age of 13.

Depression

To help them control their illness and feel healthier, certain persons with depression choose non-drug interventions. For milder symptoms of depression, natural therapies and herbal remedies can be suitable.

Depression is a chronic mood condition with signs varying from moderate to crippling and likely life-threatening.

Saffron

It is a spice from a dried part of a crocus in the iris family, an herb. According to a report in Alternative Medicine, it successfully manages mild to moderate depression by takingsaffron stigma.

Natural food retailers can advertise herbs and supplements as being able to relieve depression. However, some of these approaches have not been proven to be successful in managing depression, according to a study reported in BJ Psych Advances. This included the herbs below:

- Crataegus oxyacantha (Hawthorn)
- Ginkgo Biloba
- Eschscholzia californica (California Poppy)
- Lavandula angustifolia (Lavender)
- Melissa officinalis (Lemon Balm)
- Matricaria recutita (Chamomile)
- Passiflora incarnate (Maypop, or Purple Passionflower)
- Valeriana officinalis (Valerian)
- Piper methysticum (Kava)

Wounds

Efficient Home Remedies for Open Wounds Healing

Open wounds are indeed a nightmare; they are not only painful and messy, but they still require months to recover fully. They leave, not to overlook, a lasting stain on your skin. If it isn't enough, the wound must also be safeguarded from getting poisoned, slowing down the healing process. It may or may not encourage the wound to heal by adding various commercial ointments, but some kitchen items may work wonders. Due to their medicinal powers, some ingredients widely used in edible delicacies serve as healers or ideal cures. These natural remedies will help you to disinfect your wound. To get the most outstanding performance, make sure to use them daily. Please notice that these ingredients function well for mild wound therapies. Please resort to treatment under observation in the event of serious injuries.

Here are a few home remedies to ensure fast recovery and avoid infection.

Turmeric

The humble kitchen spice is a natural antiseptic and antibiotic product used therapeutically for years. According to research published in Molecular and Cellular Biochemistry, curcumin in turmeric helps improve wound healing by modulating collagen. Add turmeric to the wound if the wound is bleeding, and the bleeding will stop instantly. Drink a glass of milk with turmeric every night before goingto bed to fully recover.

Garlic

Garlic has been noted for its antimicrobial and antibiotic abilities, which can help stop bleeding quickly, minimize pain, and encourage healing. Currently, garlic often strengthens the standard protection of the body against infection. Just apply some crushed garlic cloves if the wound is bleeding.

Aloe Vera

The analgesic, anti-inflammatory, and relaxing effects of Aloe Vera promote the phase of recovery. In addition, there are phytochemicals in the gel that help alleviate pain and decrease inflammation. Break open the leaves of the aloe vera and remove the gel. Place the gel on the wound and allow it to dry. With warm water, rinse the region and pat dry with a towel.

Coconut Oil

Coconut oil helps relieve pain and keeps diseases at bay due to its moisturizing, antibacterial, and anti-inflammatory effects. It also helps prevent scarring. This oil must be added with a clean cloth to the infected region and covered. Then, at least 2-3 times a day, reapply. Coconut oil tends to relieve pain and keep infections at bay.

Onion

Onion does have an antimicrobial component called allicin, which prevents the wound from infection. In a mixer, mix the onion and honey and create a paste. Directly apply to the wound to speed up the process of healing.

MOST COMMON DIY HERBALRECIPES

Teas

Cold Care Tea

Ingredients:

- ¼ teaspoon sage leaves
- ¼ teaspoon calendula flower
- ¼ teaspoon elderflower
- ¼ teaspoon Hibiscus flower

Instructions:

1. Boil the water in a pot.
2. Add all the ingredients to the serving cup and mix well.
3. Pour boiling water into the serving cup with the mixture.
4. Cover the cup and steep it for 8 minutes.
5. You can mix in honey as per your taste.
6. Serve and enjoy it.

Respiratory Support Tea

Ingredients:

- ¼ teaspoon marshmallow root
- 1/3 teaspoon mullein

- ¼ teaspoon rose hips
- ¼ teaspoon lemon balm
- ¼ teaspoon
- Osha root
- ¼ teaspoon coltsfoot leaves

Instructions:

1. Boil the water in a pot.
2. Mix Osha and marshmallow roots.
3. Cover the saucepan and simmer on low heat for 10 minutes.
4. Stir in the remaining items and mix well.
5. Cover the pot and set it aside for 10 minutes to steep.
6. You can mix in honey as per your taste.
7. Strain the tea in serving cups.
8. Serve and enjoy it.

Cayenne Tea

Ingredients:

- 1/8 teaspoon cayenne powder
- One teaspoon honey
- Two teaspoons of lemon juice

Instructions:

1. Boil the water in a pot.
2. Add all the ingredients to the serving cup and mix well.
3. Pour boiling water into a serving cup with the lemon

mixture.

4. Cover the cup and steep it for 8 minutes.
5. You can mix in honey as per your taste.
6. Serve and enjoy it.

Easy Masala Tea

Ingredients:

- One teaspoon cinnamon
- One teaspoon ginger
- One teaspoon cardamom
- ½ clove
- One teaspoon of black tea leaves
- ¼ teaspoon black peppercorns
- 2 cups water
- 1 ½ cups milk

Instructions:

1. First, crush cinnamon, peppercorn, cardamom, and clove in a mortar.
2. Add water to a pan and bring it to a boil.
3. Add the crushed spices and ginger.
4. Cover the pan and reduce the flame to low.
5. Let it simmer for 20 minutes.
6. Stir in milk and tea leaves.
7. Cover the pan again and cook it for 7 minutes.
8. Remove the pan from the flame and let it steep for six more minutes.
9. You can add honey or sugar as per your taste.
10. Strain the tea in serving cups.
11. Serve and enjoy it.

Herbal Tea

Ingredients:

- 1/3 teaspoon elderberries
- 1/3 teaspoon rose hips
- 1/3 teaspoon echinacea
- 1/3 teaspoon chamomile
- 1/3 teaspoon astragals

Instructions:

1. Boil the water in a pot.
2. Add all the ingredients to the serving cup and mix well.
3. Pour boiling water into the serving cup with the mixture.
4. Cover the cup and steep it for 8 minutes.
5. You can mix in honey as per your taste.
6. Serve and enjoy it.

Decoctions

Basil Decoction

Method:

1. Boil 2 – 3 tablespoons of basil leaves in a cup of water. Steep for 10-15 minutes with a lid.
2. To make the decoction more concentrated, add more basil leaves.
3. Put your hot decoction and strain it with a strainer or cheesecloth into an empty cup.
4. Thoroughly clean up the filter if used before storing it for later use. Drink this hot herbal tea twice daily for best results.
5. Other components for your decoction include mint, rosemary, and lavender.

Also, note that rosemary can be used instead of basil for a more potent decoction.

German Chamomile Decoction

Method:

1. Boil 1 – 2 tablespoons of chamomile flowers in a cup of water. Steep for 10-15 minutes with a lid.
2. Take your hot chamomile decoction and strain it using a strainer or cheesecloth into an empty cup.
3. Thoroughly clean up the filter if used before storing it for later use. Drink this hot herbal tea twice daily for best results.
4. You may want to include other ingredients in your decoction: mint leaves, rosemary, or lavender.

Also, note that rosemary can be used instead of chamomile for a more concentrated decoction.

Chicory Decoction

Method:

1. Boil 1 – 2 tablespoons of chicory roots in a cup of water.
2. Steep for 5-10 minutes with a lid.
3. Put your hot decoction and strain it with a strainer or cheesecloth into an empty cup.
4. Thoroughly clean up the filter if used before storing it for later use.
5. Drink this hot herbal tea twice daily for best results.

You may want to include other ingredients in your decoction: mint leaves, rosemary, or lavender.

Ginger Decoction

Method:

1. Boil 1 – 2 tablespoons of ginger in a cup of water.
2. Steep for 10-15 minutes with a lid.
3. Put your hot decoction and strain it with a strainer or cheesecloth into an empty cup.
4. Thoroughly clean up the filter if used before storing it for later use.
5. Drink this hot herbal tea twice daily for best results.
6. You may want to include other ingredients in your decoction: mint leaves, rosemary, or lavender.

Ginkgo Berry Decoction

Method:

1   1 – 2 tablespoons of Ginkgo in a cup of water.
2   Steep for 10-15 minutes with a lid.
3   Put your hot decoction and strain it with a strainer or cheesecloth into an empty cup.
4   Thoroughly clean up the filter if used before storing it for later use. Drink this hot herbal tea twice daily for best results.

You may want to include other ingredients in your decoction: mint leaves, rosemary, or lavender.

Ice Cubes

Ice cubes are a fantastic source of herbal delivery and are straightforward to administer. They can be made from teas and decoctions as well. Liquid herbal medicine can be frozen after boiling and have a rapid cooling in a process called thawing. It also contains pain-relieving benefits, which are very specific to cold therapy. If we add sticks inside ice cubes, they can easily be turned into homemade sweet popsicles. This form of administration is highly famous among children. The ice bags and trays should be labeled accordingly to avoid issues.

Baths

Lavender Bath

Preparation:

1. Add 1 to 2 cups of dried lavender flower to your bathtub. Boil a pot of water and add 1/2 cup of Epsom salt.
2. Pour the liquid into the bathtub, then get in when the water has been added.
3. Soak for 5 to 10 minutes.

Use with caution because the Epsom salt may irritate those who are sensitive to it.

Sage Bath

Preparation:

1. Place 1/4 cup of dried sage in your bathtub and add

hot water. Steep for 5 to 10 minutes before
gettinginto the tub.
2. For extra effect, you can leave the herbs in the tub
    after your bath.

It is recommended not to use this herbal treatment if you are
pregnant or breastfeeding because sage has properties that
can make you feel like you're on an intense trip.

Rose Petal Bath

Preparation:

1. Place 8 to 10 organic rose petals into your bathtub.
2. Vitamin C in rose petals brightens and softens skin.
3. Steep the rose petals in hot water for 3 to 5
    minutes before getting into the tub.

Rose glyceride is a substance in rose petals that can soothe
irritations and inflammation caused by eczema and acne.

Ginger Bath

Ginger is an essential element in improving your skin's
health. The best ginger is fresh ginger, which can be added
to your bath as a decoction or powder.

If you make the decoction, use two parts of water for one
part of ginger root.

Preparation:

1. Add 1/2 cup of Epsom salt and 1 cup of fresh
    ginger root for each other.
2. Use 3 to 4 cups of hot water for each person taking a

bath. Steep in a pot for 5-10 minutes.
3. When ready to take a bath, use 1/2 cup of the mixture with the Epsom salt and add it to your bathwater.
4. Soak for 5-10 minutes before rinsing.

Precautions: do not use this herbal treatment if you have high blood pressure because ginger can increase blood pressure levels. Also, do not take this herbal bath if you are pregnant.

Breast Milk

Lemon Balm

Lemon balm has been found to help infants with colic, fussiness, and other digestive problems. It has also been known to soothe infant fussiness and relieve cramps. Also has been demonstrated in studies to help boost breast milk supply and increase nutrients in the milk of nursing moms.

Method:

1. Add 1/4 teaspoon of finely ground lemon balm powder or 2 to 3 drops of lemon balm essential oil to 4 ounces of breastmilk.
2. Warm the breast milk either by the microwave or on the stove. Serve it to your baby.
3. Repeat every two hours during the day and as needed for relief.

Do not use this herbal treatment if the mother is breastfeeding a preterm infant.

Chamomile

Chamomile is a common herbal remedy for treating children's colic, fever, and teething. It is known to help reduce swelling, soothe irritable newborns, and relieve fevers. Chamomile can also be used for making herbal infant teas or tinctures.

Method:

1. Add 1/4 teaspoon of finely ground chamomile or

2 to 3 drops of chamomile essential oil to 4
ounces of breastmilk.

2. Warm the breast milk either by the microwave or on
   the stove. Serve it to your baby.
3. Repeat every two hours during the day and as
   needed for relief.

Do not use this herbal treatment if the mother is
breastfeeding a preterm infant.

Calendula

Calendula is also known as marigold. It can be used to make
herbal teas for infants or be added to a bath in a bit of water.
In addition, Calendula has strong anti-inflammatory
properties.

Method:

1. Add 1/4 teaspoon of finely ground calendula or
   2 to 3 drops of calendula essential oil to 4 ounces
   of breast milk.
2. Arm the breast milk either by the microwave or on
   the stove. Serve it to your baby.
3. Repeat every two hours during the day and as
   needed for relief.

Do not use this herbal treatment if the mother is
breast feeding a preterm infant.

Washcloths

Eyewash

Preparation:

1. Add a few drops of water into the eye spray bottle.
2. Fill the rest of the bottle with peppermint essential oil. Use these eye drops to clean the eye area.

This is very good for people who suffer from dry eyes, as they can treat them with one quick and simple wash. Refrigerate in an airtight container after each use to ensure potency. The eyewash can also be used for other purposes, such as treating conjunctivitis, blepharitis, and other eye issues.

Tongue Wash

Preparation:

1. Fill the tongue spray bottle with water.
2. Fill the rest of the bottle with thyme essential oil.
3. Use this tongue spray to clean the area around the mouth, and in its presence, you will feel a soothing sensation on your tongue.
4. This is an excellent treatment if you have bad breath and provides cleanliness to the inside of your mouth. After usage, please keep it in an airtight container for two weeks.
5. This tongue wash can be used on other body parts such as the inner thigh area, groin area, armpit, and any other areas that may need a light cleaning and soothing. Armpit Wash Preparation:

6. Fill the armpit spray bottle with a few drops of water. Add lavender essential oil to the bottle.
7. Use this armpit spray to clean your armpits, and you will feel a soothing sensation on your skin.
8. This is very good for people who work in the construction field, as it will help remove odors from the body and develop an antibacterial treatment for skin infections. In an airtight container, it lasts two weeks.
9. The armpit wash can also be used on other body areas such as the groin area, inner thigh area, and back of the neck to get a good cleaning.

Poultices

Herbal Healing Salve

Ingredients:
- 1 cup calendula almond oil
- 1/3 cup beeswax
- 1 cup comfrey almond oil
- 1 teaspoon essential oil of rose geranium
- ½ cup plantain-infused almond oil
- 8 tablespoons of herbal mixture

Instructions:

1. Add the herb mixture to the jar and pour over the almond oil.
2. Close the lid and shake well.
3. For at least 65 days, keep the jar in a warm environment.
4. Strain the oil from the mixture using cheesecloth and discard the solids of the mix.
5. Store at a dark place. The infused oil for the salve is ready.
6. Now add water to a pot and let it boil.
7. Add beeswax to a small pan and place it over boiling water to melt the wax.
8. When the wax is melted, add the infused oils and stir well.
9. Remove the pan from the boiling water and set it aside.
10. It will take a few hours to cool down.
11. The healing salve is ready to use.

Herbal Poultice

Ingredients:

- One teaspoon of turmeric powder
- Two teaspoons of coconut oil
- One cup sliced onion
- One teaspoon garlic
- Four tablespoons of ginger paste

Instructions:

1. Combine all the ingredients in a pan and cook over low flame until the content gets dry.
2. Remove the pan from the flame and let it stand for a while.
3. Transfer the mixture to the cheesecloth, then fold and tie the cloth.
4. Massage the affected area with the pouch for about 30 minutes.
5. This poultice is used as an anti-inflammatory agent.

Bran Poultice

Ingredients:

- Water
- Bran

Instructions:

1. Add water to a pot and boil it.
2. Add bran and mix well to form a paste.
3. Apply while hot on the affected area.

4. This poultice can be used to relieve strains, bruises, and inflammation.

Mustard Poultice

Ingredients:

- Mustard powder
- Water
- Flour

Instructions:

1. Add mustard powder to water and make a paste.
2. Use flour to thicken the paste.
3. Add in a cloth and massage.
4. It can be used to treat arthritis and improve circulation.

Bread Poultice

Ingredients:

- Bread & Milk

Instructions:

1. In a pot, heat the milk over medium fire. Keep it aside to cool down a little. Add bread slices and let them stand in the warm milk.
2. Mix bread with the milk to form a paste. Now, apply over the skin and leave it for about 20 minutes. You can use it on a cyst, splinter, and abscess.

Tinctures

Indigestion Tincture

Preparation:

1. Combine one tablespoon of dried mint leaves in a pot with a half cup of water.
2. Please bring it to a boil, remove it from the heat and let it sit for 10 minutes to soak and cool.
3. Line the alembic with cheesecloth, and then add the mint mixture through it into your bottle of choice.
4. Now, screw the cap on firmly and store it in a cool and dark place for at least two weeks.
5. Take two spoonsful of tincture into the mouth and swish it around to spread it evenly on your teeth, gums, and other parts of your mouth.
6. After that, you can take more tinctures depending on how well you feel after the first application.
7. You can also add the tincture to your food or juices.

Cough and Cold Tincture

Preparation:

1. Mix one tablespoon of chamomile with one cup of water in a pot.
2. Boil the mixture for about five minutes and then cover it until cooled for at least ten minutes.
3. Use 2-3 drops of tincture as needed for cough or cold. This tincture unlocks bactericidal powers.

Painkiller Tincture

Preparation:

1. Six one tablespoon of Chamomile with two cups of water in a pot.
2. Oil the mixture for about five minutes and then cover it until cooled for at least ten minutes.
3. Use 2-3 drops of tincture as needed for headaches, cramps, or other types of pain.

Infusions

Sore Throat Infusion

Preparation:

1. Fill a pot halfway with water, add one teaspoon of fresh ginger, and bring it to a boil.
2. Allow 10 minutes to steep after turning off the burner.
3. Use 1-2 teaspoons of the mixture as often as needed for sore throat pain relief.

People who regularly take this infusion, including the sage and fennel, have fewer cases of sore throat yearly because they have solid bacterial resistance.

Infusion of Sage

Preparation:

1. Pour two cups of water into a pot, add one ounce of sage leaves and bring it to a boil.
2. Allow 10 minutes to steep after turning off the burner.
3. Use 2-4 teaspoons of the mixture as often as needed for chest colds.

Infusion of Fennel

Preparation:

1. Fill a pot halfway with water, add one teaspoon of fresh ginger, and bring it to a boil.
2. Allow 10 minutes to steep after turning off the burner.

3. Use 1-2 teaspoons of the mixture as often as needed for cold, cough, and respiratory disorders.

People who regularly take this infusion have fewer cases of constipation every year

Infusion of Valerian

Preparation:

- Pour two cups of water into a pot, add one teaspoon of fresh parsley flowers, and bring it to a boil.
- Allow 10 minutes to steep after turning off the burner.
- Use 2-4 teaspoons with ½ teaspoon of valerian root for insomnia, anxiety, and nervousness.

People who regularly take this infusion have fewer cases of insomnia every year.

Infusion of Yellow Dock Tea

Preparation:

1. Fill a pot halfway with water, add one teaspoon of fresh ginger, and bring it to a boil.
2. Allow 10 minutes to steep after turning off the burner.
3. se 1-2 teaspoons for liver disorders, skin problems, and urinary tract infections.

People who regularly take this infusion have fewer liver disorders and skin problems yearly because of the strong bacterial resistance it provides.

ABOUT HERB SUPPLY

Growing Your Herbs

Growing herbs is a terrific way to add color and flavor to your yard, but it can also be simple and easy if done correctly. Tons of herbs can be grown indoors in pots on your windowsill, but some also need a bit more work to grow well. However, no matter what herb you want, some things makelife easier when grown indoors, and others don't.

The first thing you should do is plant your herbs. It's easy to grow them in some containers but if you want to get the most out of your pots, choose herbs that require more water or humidity. You can also use bigger pots but make sure they're at least 4 inches deep (or more) and at least 9 inches across (or more).

To keep your herbs healthy, keep them away from direct sunlight, and if you can put them out on the ground partially during the day, even better. If you don't have a sunny windowsill, try placing the pots on a table or shelf in front ofa south-facing window.

When choosing which herb to grow, consider what it's good for and, of course, the smell. For instance, you can grow basil and cilantro to make your food taste better, repel foul odors and flies, and even keep yourself healthy. You might even want to keep a plant of each kind.

Some herbs need more water than others, so it's best to be informed about this before you start growing them. For instance, chives don't need as much water as parsley or mint (this depends on the variety you choose). However, they'll wilt or mold if they get too much water.

It's also essential to grow the same herb every year, but you can use different pots in different containers. For example, keep some herbs in small pots and others in bigger containers.

To grow your herbs indoors, you'll need either a herb pot for each plant or a pot big enough for all your plants (or you can buy 4-10). It would help if you also put drainage holes in the bottom of the pool. The holes should be around 1/4" wide and 1/4" deep to allow proper drainage.

Before putting your plants in their pots, make sure to soak them in water (if needed) and ensure they're dried before planting them. This will eliminate the risk of them moldingor wilting.

When it comes to watering, if your herbs are in pots, make sure they get water every day (or every other day) and if you keep them in their final pots, make sure they get poured with plenty of water (enough to fill the entire pot). Also, make sure that the soil receives watered enough.

Advice on Buying Herbs

I understand that not anyone has access to a forest or a meadow near their home, so I decided to write this paragraph as a guide to the conscious purchase of herbs.

Although you may find the herbs you need for your preparations in the grocery store or herbal shop, my advice is to rely on local producers, they may be more expensive, but the quality is higher and generally worth the price.

When purchasing herbs, you must look at three key factors to determine the quality:

Soil: ask where the herbs have been cultivated and research the country's regulations regarding pollution. This task may seem complicated, but many big retailers already offer this certification of conformity in their products. If you are interested in urban farms, ask them if they use clean soil and if they have water filtration systems

Growing Practices: The aspects you must take care of when inquiring about growing practices are fertilizers, insect management, and outdoor/greenhouse/hydroponic cultivation.

Drying: Drying temperature is critical. If too high, it will burn the leaves, and you will lose all their precious substances. Also, look at the color of the leaves and discard them if it isbrown-black.

My go-to advice, in this case, is to trust your senses. If the herbs have vivid color and give off a fragrant aroma, their quality is almost certainly good.

Being someone who wildcrafts and dries her herbs, I have found the sweet spot is a temperature between 77°F and 86°F in a dark environment with the plants widely spaced or hung upside down from the ceiling. I found that leaves and flowers are dehydrated in roughly one week and roots in one month using these low temperatures. Of course, real drying times depend on the plant itself, its water percentage, and the size, so I always recommend checking if leaves and flowers are "crunchy" and if roots are dry on the inside by cutting a sample.

Wild Crafting

Many people who explore herbalism for the first time, or those specifically interested in Native American Herbalism, are probably wondering what wildcrafting is. The answer is simple: it is a method of harvesting medicinal herbs from areas humans have not cleared or cultivated.

Wildcrafting is a term that encompasses gathering plants from the wilds of Earth. This herbalism is often associated with Native Americans forced to adapt to their homeland's light conditions.

Wildcrafting is a term that refers to gathering plant seeds and berries for nutritional and medicinal purposes; the practice was introduced to the world by the Native Americans, who used it as a food source and medicine for their families.

Wildcrafting can be challenging to do. It involves locating patches of plants deep within forests or hillsides far away from roads with trails and other disturbances like hikers and campfires. Foragers must often know a good deal about native plants before they head into such environments because some can be poisonous if misidentified and consumed. Learning to identify a particular plant species and its specific parts is essential before attempting to harvest from it.

Many people will go outside into their local environment, go hiking through different natural areas, or look for herbs in their backyards if they are interested in wildcrafting. It will help them become familiar with the plants growing there to learn, potentially beneficial for medicinal purposes. In addition, many people who want to know about wildcrafting have found it more accessible than they initially thought since many resources are available with maps of different regions that show where certain herbs grow.

CONCLUSION

Native American herbal remedies are a standard alternative treatment used throughout the United States for centuries. The practice involves taking natural plant extracts to treat a particular ailment.

The best place to start looking for these remains is Native-American-herbal- remedies.com, which provides detailed information on their creation and properties. There is also a list of some of the most common illnesses that can be treated through herbs, like diabetes, eczema, and more! They're easy to use and often have favorable side effects; it'shard not to get excited about them.

Most of these remedies have been passed down through the generations and are often used traditionally in Apache, Haida, Navajo, and other Native American communities. They can be ingested in pill form or used topically in the form of tea or salves. Some contain no active ingredients at all but do have a positive impact on one's system.

These remedies could be used for various reasons, like treating diabetes and asthma (as well as conditions in non-native Americans). Still, many people choose them for their mood-boosting properties as well. In addition, it is said that many herbal remedies have stress-reducing qualities, which can help treat issues like mood swings and anxiety. And, if all else fails, there's always traditional counseling or medication.

There are several advantages of using herbs. First, they're

natural, so there's no chance of overdosing and adverse side effects. Plus, they contain very little that could be absorbed in large quantities, which makes them safe to take.

One problem with many types of drugs is that they can damage cell receptors in your body—a process called receptor desensitization. This is one of the main reasons people, after surgery or recovery, tend to get sick more easily as their immune systems are not yet fully active. But with herbal remedies, this isn't a concern.

They also hit the body in a particular and targeted way, another advantage many drugs do not possess. An example of this is St. John's wort, which

helps with many mood-related issues by promoting feelings of calmness and happiness. Many people use it to relieve symptoms of depression, seasonal affective disorder (SAD), or anxiety—but they all have very different ways of doing so,thanks to their different chemical compositions.

As with any alternative treatment or medication, there are some potential drawbacks. For example, the long-term effects of these herbal remedies have not been studied enough to know their implications. They could have side effects, or they might cause complications.

It is also important to note that Native-American-herbal-remedies.com provides a list of these remedies and the best ways to use them properly, but that isn't comprehensive. However, it is beneficial to understand what they can do and how they work.

Overall, the main reason why these herbal remedies are used

is that they're effective. Many people swear by them and use them to treat all kinds of conditions, and there are no recorded instances of lousy side effects. That alone provides a lot of weight in favor of using them for many different reasons.

NATIVE AMERICAN HERBAL RECIPES

INTRODUCTION

Native American Herbs are an ancestral gift of nature to Native Americans and are often used in healing, spiritual, and everyday life and can be found in many different classes. These resources will help increase understanding of how they can improve well-being. In addition, a plethora of information about herbs can help with physical and psychological well-being.

A plant has been grown for hundreds of years and has natural properties that make it a suitable medicine. Herbs are the foundation of food, treatment, and everyday living. They provide health benefits from the simple to the powerful ones. Our ancestors recognized these natural qualities and used these herbs to promote wellness, vitality, and longevity.

The roots, leaves, barks, flowers, or seeds of a plant can be brought together to make a type of liquid medicine called tincture or syrup that you or your family can use.

Modern science is figuratively using the same practices our ancestors did thousands (or perhaps millions) of years ago to extract valuable medicines from plants.

Today's scientists use the same knowledge that Native Americans and ancestors used to make herbal medicines. In many cases, these medicines can be stronger than the originalplant employed to make them.

The following information will provide you with herbal remedies for conditions you may have or are experiencing, such as cancer, heart disease, weight loss, weight gain, and so much more. It will also teach you how to use herbs in your everyday life to improve energy and take care of your health.

Plants and herbs come in many forms, such as leaves, barks, roots, buds, flowers, and seeds. Each has its healing properties but do they have to be used together?

None of these four categories of plants and herbs (leaves, barks, roots, and flowers) are better than the other concerning healing. Each category contains distinct set of chemical ingredients that enable it to be beneficial in improving health.

The Leaves category is the herbs that can be combined with the ones mentioned above. These plants can be used for their known healing properties of improving or enhancing health and maintaining wellness.

The next category is the Barks Class; these can be used to treat a wide variety of conditions and ailments that your body may be experiencing. From cancer to weight loss, a wide range of conditions can be treated using barks and other similar plants.

Next, we have the Roots category. These herbs are known to have health benefits when they are ingested. They can help alleviate symptoms of various conditions and, in some cases, restore health.

Another group is the Flowers category. These herbs can promote wellness or enhance your well-being depending on conditions and ailments you may have. A wide range of medicinal uses could be seen from this class of plants, especially if you have a need that is not improving or maintaining wellness.

We can also find the Seeds category. These seeds have a wide range of healing properties that can be ingested to treat many ailments and conditions. From reversing aging to helping with cancer, these plants have been proven effective in enhancing well-being.

Now you may wonder about the herb's proper use; let's see some frequently asked questions about this.

What is the difference between fresh or dried herbs? Fresh herbs are preferred for making herbal remedies because their properties are more potent than dried herbs when appropriately prepared. However, freshness counts for many of the active chemical compounds found in most herbs and plants will diminish over time because of exposure to light, heat, and air.

Are herbs safe for children? Many safe herbs can be used to treat ailments in children. Some of these herbs may also be useful for adults. The herbs in the following lines are safe for children and adults.

MEDICINAL PLANTS USED DAILY BY NATIVE AMERICANS

Butterbur (Petasites)

Butterbur, also known as Petasites, is another medicinal herb found in the Pacific North West. It has extensive underground rhizomes and is a perennial. It can also be identified by its leaves which are rhubarb-like. Parts of this plant that are usable for medicinal purposes include the roots, leaves, and stems.

Mullein (Verbascum)

Mullein is a perennial plant that grows to around 3 meters tall. Its leaves are soft, hairy, and arranged in a spiral manner. The flowers are yellow and appear atop the plant, giving it a unique appearance. The parts of this plant that are of medicinal value are the leaves and flowers.

Oat Seed (Avena Sativa)

Nervine tonic is another name for oat seed because of its significant impact on mental health; this is an excellent plant used to treat symptoms of fatigue and stress related to the brain's health. Another benefit of this plant is using it against many addictions, including nicotine and cannabis.

Green Tea (Camellia Sinensis)

Tea is well known and probably the most consumed beverage in the world. The use of this herb for medicinal purposes is well general and has a strong research background. Black tea requires the essential and partial fermentation process of the tea leaves. However, green tea doesn't need these kinds of fermentation and can be produced by steaming the leaves. This process reduces the oxidation capacities of enzymes in tea leaves, and the preservation of polyphenol is achieved through this process.

Devil's Club (Oplopanax Horridus)

This plant belongs to the ginseng family, and botanically, it is considered in the Araliaceae family. Therefore, another name implied to this plant is Devil stick or Devil's walking cane. Its roots, leaves, and stem are used for herbal medicinal purposes.

Alfalfa (Medicago Sativa)

Alfalfa is a very cleansing digestive detoxifier for the gut. Research has observed Alfalfa binding to carcinogens in the colon. European studies suggest that the regular consumption of Alfalfa helps lower cholesterol.

Arnica (Arnica Montana)

A sunny healer for bruises, muscle aches, sprains, and arthritis. Use the dried flower heads in oils, salves, or tinctures for applying to the skin where muscles, bones, or joints are sore. Or, visit your local natural food or medicine section—Arnica creams and ointments are popular!

Black Haw (Viburnum Prunifolium)

This beautiful bush—with bright red berries and cream-colored flowers—is a cornerstone favorite in the United States Southern herbalism. It was once used for all sorts of women's health issues by Native Americans, even for childbirth, miscarriage, and labor.

Now, it has settled into the comfortable role of allaying uterine cramps that come with menstruation—but anyone, man or woman, can enjoy its ability to take away intestinal or stomach cramps.

Black Cohosh (Actaea Racemosa)

Native to North America, this stunning plant (once used for snakebites in Native herbalism) has become a critical herbal medicine for women today; it contains "phytoestrogens," which mimic estrogen and fit perfectly in females hormone receptors.

Boneset (Eupatorium Perfoliaturn)

It might be hard not to think this plant has something to do with bones. But its ancient, old-time use was for alleviating colds, flu, and fevers so intense that they made your bones hurt!

Prepare the dried leaves of this tall plant in a hot tea or tincture, and take them daily during minor viral illnesses.

Cinnamon (Cinnamomum Zeylonicum)

Sweet spice for sweet problems: diabetes and cholesterol. Ironically, this spice commonly found with sweet foods happens to be excellent at blood sugar control. Cinnamon is the sweet, powdered inner bark residue from mighty evergreen trees native to India and China. Cinnamon essential oils are available but should not be used internally. Supplements of Cinnamon are available, though it can, of course, be used in meals and even in a tea or tincture at home.

Elder (Sambucus Nigra)

Esteemed virus-fighter and fever supporter of the herb world. If you were to combine echinacea, boneset, and ginger, you would have an entirely natural herbal medicine to combat any cold or flu that comes your way. Add elder, and all your bases are covered! This vivid, dark purple berry is delicious, stimulates the immune system, and combats viruses. Dried elderberries make a delightful tea or infusion and a tasty tincture.

Eucalyptus (Eucalyptus Globulus)

Australia's premier herb for respiratory healing. A stunning Aussie tree is now found worldwide; Eucalyptus has snuck its way into many over-the- counter cough medicines—maybe without us realizing we depend on plant healing already! Oils in the leaves are antibacterial, antiviral, and anti- inflammatory, but the plant is incredibly best at opening up the lungs and assisting with coughs. Seek eucalyptus in essential oils and supplements. In addition, dried leaves are available to make teas, tinctures, salves, and oils for healing.

Evening Primrose (Oenothera Biennis)

An herbal source for Omega-3 and inflammation soothing. Because it blooms in the evening, Evening primrose is given a unique, mysterious name. Its benefits are not so mysterious, though—high amounts of plant mucilage contain Omega-3 fatty acids, making it a target in the herbal world for dealing with inflammatory issues. Evening primrose is active only in oil form

—look for oil capsules or topical oils at natural food stores. If you are an advanced herbalist, try making your sun-infused oil of the seed pods.

Goldenseal (Hydrastis Canadensis)

Nature's magic, natural antibiotic, and digestive tonic. Goldenseal's use originated among the Native Americans, who then introduced it to English settlers. Today, it has achieved study and reputation enough to be one of the most wildly popular herbs—though it does hold an endangered status. Traditional and mainstream medicine uphold it as an antibiotic and healer of numerous digestive issues. Use the dried root to make a (very bitter) tea, tincture, ointment, or salve. Supplements are available—topical use can help with skin and digestive infections.

Milk Thistle (Silybum Marianum)

A one-of-a-kind liver herb—unparalleled in modern

medicine. Rarely is there a plant out there that can achieve what mainstream medications cannot, and milk thistle is the exception. It is a prickly plant, but the seeds have certain powers on the liver. It might be just the healer for those experiencing liver issues. One can make a tea of the seeds as a home remedy. Milk thistle supplements are readily available at most stores in capsule form.

Motherwort (Leonurus Cardiac)

A heart-warming ally for cardiovascular health. Some may plague Motherwort as a noxious weed with spiny, irritating burrs that attach to your clothes. Little do they know; a preparation of leaves and flowers could be one of the most beautiful natural heart tonics out there! Make and use your homemade tea or tincture if you desire. Motherwort supplements are not uncommon either and are an option at natural food grocers.

Nettles (Urtica Dioica)

Keeping those non-flowering, seedless nettle tops might make for an incredibly nutritious supplement or relief for allergies. Pick with gloves, hang, and dry for 1 hour to remove the sting. Use a tincture or supplement for allergy and urinary issues or cook greens from Nettle tops before they flower. Pot for a thick infusion of the leaves for Nettle's nutritional content, excellent for the anemic or malnourished.

Plantain (Plantago)

Plantain is a ubiquitous herb found practically everywhere in the world. Once upon a time, it was revered as a cleansing, cancer-fighting folk remedy— there's no evidence of that, but today it holds the trophy as a digestive tonic, laxative, and topical wound healer. Incorporate plantain into oils and salves for topical use, or consider a piping hot tea for bowel irregularities.

Rosemary (Rosmarinus Officinalis)

Rosemary is probably more well-known for perking up roasted vegetables and Mediterranean dishes. But its history of addition to foods is not only for taste—its antioxidant capabilities were so powerful that they prevented foods from oxidizing and going rancid. In addition, those same antioxidant capabilities can be excellent for age-fighting, while other compounds can kill bacteria, improve circulation, and reduce inflammation.

Reishi (Ganoderma tsugae)

Reishi contains polysaccharides and triterpenes, which modulate the immune system's creation of inflammation. It can thus help with the pain and management of auto-immune disorders—like Rheumatoid Arthritis or Lupus.

Tea Tree (Melaleuca Alternifolia)

The herbal world's skin healer, cleanser, and protector. The Tea Tree's power as an antimicrobial is almost unrivaled among herbs. Originating from Australia (like Eucalyptus), it is now a standard herbal product, especially for skin issuesand wounds.

Thyme (Thymus Vulgaris)

Much like Eucalyptus and Mint, Thyme has snuck its way into many an over-the-counter cold and flu remedy; this is probably because this culinary herb also has bronchial-dilating, decongestant, expectorant, and antimicrobial powers. Make a tea of the sprigs, or keep your tincture for use at home. It's also a popular essential oil for topical use and a healing supplement for internal use.

FOUR INCREDIBLE THINGS HERBAL REMEDIES CAN DO

Herbal remedies continue to increase in popularity. As a result, more and more people choose to benefit from these natural remedies to treat their ailments and protect their health. According to the World Health Organization (WHO), herbal medicines are used by around 80% of the world's population for health purposes. However, you may not yet know about some of these things, and your physician may never tell you about the other facts.

More Affordable Treatment

Using herbs as natural remedies enable you to save your hard-earned money. Saving money may not be possible with pharmaceutical medicines, given their typically high cost. Aside from being the more affordable solution for ailments, botanical remedies are equally effective as drug-based medications.

The Harvard Medical School recognizes the ability of botanicals to heal. It has published a special health report on treating common pain conditions without using drugs or surgery. In addition, several studies and research show that plant-based medications work well with the body systems.

Safer Treatment than Drugs

Herbs and other natural remedies are safer treatments than drug-based medicines. Typically, herbal medicines do not carry side effects because of their natural composition. On the other hand, drugs contain active ingredients that interferewith the body systems, hence, the side effects.

Side effects of pharmaceutical medicines often occur (a) when you start taking the medication, (b) change the dosage, to lower it or strengthen it, and (c) when you stop taking your medicine(s). In contrast, the side effects of herbal treatments are generally attributable to improper use.

Similar Potency to Pharmaceuticals

At first glance, herbal medicines may not be as potent as pharmaceutical medicines when comparing their dosage. For instance, a cup of willow bark tea (naturally containing aspirin and acting as a pain reliever) is weaker than the standard dosage of pharmaceutical aspirin.

However, instead of looking at the dosage comparison, look at the effects of these medications. If taking a cup of willow bark can suffice to relieve your pain, why risk your general health to the typical side effects of pharmaceutical medicines? Instead, consider a general rule in medication, and start taking your treatment with the lowest dosage possible.

More Effective Treatment for Chronic Conditions

Treating chronic conditions is no longer as difficult as it once was. Many available treatments can make the symptoms of certain diseases much more bearable. However, for those who would like to avoid surgery or other forms of invasive surgery, there are other options as well. Chronic conditions should never be taken lightly, but with the help of a skilled team at a reliable medical clinic can often be treated and managed without surgery.

Sinusitis has been a condition that has plagued many for years, often rendering them incapacitated for weeks. Surgery is sometimes the only option when it comes to addressing sinusitis symptoms. There is, however, a new type of treatment that allows people to avoid invasive surgery while also helping them to recuperate faster than they would with past therapies; this is known as Sinuvil, and it works on patients in a way that few other treatments can. It uses a series of natural enzymes to treat inflammation within the nasal cavities and sinus passages.

Psoriasis is another chronic condition that affects millions of people each year. Fortunately, some available treatments can help alleviate psoriasis symptoms so patients can move on with their lives. One of the most effective treatments for this condition is Lupron, which uses a synthetic version of a natural hormone with some key differences. This is injected into the joints and helps to control any issues that have to do with joint or mobility issues.

Another chronic condition that many people face each year is asthma. While asthma can be managed by prescribed medication, sometimes patients would instead take alternative medicines to avoid taking the drugs, which often come with side effects. The most effective asthma treatment is known as the nebulizer. This form of therapy uses ultrasonic technology to disperse medication into the air. The drug enters the lungs, where the body can then absorb it.

Many people do not think they are in danger of developing a chronic condition because they have it under control. Still, specific events or circumstances may cause them to break down again. When this occurs, it usually indicates a blockage or obstruction within the body that requires surgical removal. However, in some cases, a less invasive option can easily be picked up and used as an alternative treatment for these patients who would instead not undergo invasive surgery.

The most common chronic conditions are arthritis and diabetes. Arthritis is a common ailment that can be treated with various methods, including medication, surgery, and chemotherapy. Diabetes is a disease that affects millions of individuals throughout the world, and it can typically be managed with diabetes medication and dietary changes. Stress can also sometimes cause the body to break down so it cannot function like it was used to. The most effective therapy for this condition is Bio-Acupuncture, and unlike mass medication, it will not have any side effects on the patient.

Botanicals, on the other hand, have no side effects or minimal side effects only. As mentioned earlier, the side effects typically occur only with improper use or dosage. In addition, herbs contain natural chemicals that can sufficiently address chronic health conditions without the risk of side effects.

HERBAL RECIPES

Used for:

Vitamin C Pills

Vitamin C tablets help to boost the immune system and fight off colds and flu-like symptoms.

Ingredients:

- One tablespoon of rose hip powder (the fruit of a rose plant, which has a high Vitamin C content)
- One tablespoon of amla powder (an Indian gooseberry that has strong antibacterial properties)
- One tablespoon acerola powder (a Barbados cherry, which is excellent for stomach discomfort)
- Honey
- Orange peel powder (optional) (orange is a citrus fruit, and its peel is often used for flavor)

Directions:

1. Blend the powdered herbs, smoothing out any clumped powder. Pour a few droplets of slightly warmed honey into the powdered mix. Stir, add a few more droplets, and stir again. Mix until the combination holds together without being too sticky

or moist.

2. Shape the mix into pea-size balls. Roll these around in the orange powder if you've selected to use it. The mixture should make 45 balls. Store these in an

airtight container to give them an extended shelf life. Take 1-3 daily.

Hyssop Oxymel

Used for:

Great for colds, flu, and bronchitis.

Ingredients:

- Hyssop, fresh or dried (an herbaceous plant with antiseptic and expectorant properties)
- Honey
- Apple cider vinegar (vinegar made from cider that is great for weight loss and heart health)

Directions:

1. Fill a jar lightly with chopped fresh hyssop. (Only half fill it if you're using dried hyssop).
2. Then, fill the jar with honey just 1/3 of the way, and top it off with the apple cider vinegar.
3. Let it sit in the sealed jar for 2-4 weeks before straining.
4. You can take 1-2 teaspoons of this remedy every hour for a congested cough. Keep the hyssop oxymel in thefridge for better preservation.

Oat Straw Infusion

Used for:

This oat straw infusion is excellent for its calming, stress-relieving effect.

Ingredients:

- Oat straw herb (comes from Avena sativa, which has long-lasting energy effects)
- Boiling water

Directions:

1. Put the oat straw into a 1-quart jar, then pour boiling water over the herb. Finally, cap it with an airtight lid.
2. Allow the mix to rest for 4-6 hours, infusing the minerals throughout the solution.
3. Strain it. You can add a little extra lavender, lemon verbena, rosemary, or other herbs to the combination once it's made if you want to.
4. Oat straw can be used as a base for juices, lemonades, and frozen concentrates. In addition, you can use it to create ice cubes or ice pops if you want a variation.

Lemon Balm Home Remedy

Used for:

Perfect for cold sore sufferers as a natural way to help prevent and eliminate the virus's effects.

Ingredients:

- Two teaspoons of lemon balm, dried (alternate: 2 lemon balm teabags)
- 1 cup water, boiled

Directions:

1. Boil water, then steep the lemon balm for 10-15 minutes. Strain.
2. Apply the mixture immediately to the cold sore using a wet cotton ball. Use it at least four times daily. Alternately, try consuming a couple of cups of tea daily to help expel the virus.

Meadowsweet Elixir

Used for:

This is a fantastic home remedy for pain relief.

Ingredients:

- 100 g meadowsweet flowers (a European flower that is known as "the stomach corrector")
- 40 ml 50% vodka (a distilled alcoholic drink that consists primarily of water and ethanol)
- 100 ml glycerin (a sugar-alcohol compound often used in elixirs and skin care products)

Directions:

1. Place the meadowsweet flowers in a jar and add the vodka and glycerin. Shake well and let it macerate for 4-6 weeks.
2. Check the mixture often, as sometimes the flowers will soak up the alcohol and glycerin so that the liquid no longer covers the herb. In this case, you either need to use a stone to weigh them down or add more alcohol.
3. After 4-6 weeks, you must strain the mixture to be ready for use.

Elderberry Gummy Bears

Used for:

These vitamin C treats are suitable for an immune system-boosting treat that looks after your well-being.

Ingredients:
- 50 g elderberries, dried
- 30 g rosehips, dried
- 15 g cinnamon chips
- 7 g licorice root
- 0.5 g pepper, freshly ground (a flowering vine, which is often used for seasoning)
- 3 cups apple cider
- Three tablespoons of gelatin (derived from collagen and used as gelling agent in food)

Directions:
1. Place all ingredients (except the gelatin) into a medium-size saucepan. Bring the mixture to simmer and continue for 20 minutes. Strain and squeeze well to extract the juice.
2. Measure 2 cups of juice (add more apple cider to make the mixture fill 2 cups). Put 1/2 cup into the fridge, then dust the gelatin on top of it after it's chilled. Allow this to sit for one minute.
3. Bring the rest of the mixture to a simmer. Combine the hot juice with the cooled gelatin mixture. Stir quickly with a whisk. Continue to mix until the gelatin is completely dissolved. If you want to sweeten this up more, add sugar or honey.
4. Pour this mixture into molds and refrigerate. They are ready to eat after they solidify. Eat 1-3 gummies

daily, and keep them in a sealed container in the
fridge.

Bitter Digestive Pastilles

Used for:

For those who suffer bitter deficiency syndrome or for promoting a healthy digestive system

Ingredients:

- 1/2 teaspoon angelica root powder (a European herb used for gastrointestinal tract disorders)
- 1/4 teaspoon gentian root powder (grows in Alpine habitats and treats digestive issues)
- 1/4 teaspoon coriander powder (great for promoting healthy digestion)
- 1/4 teaspoon orange peel powder & 1/8 teaspoon black pepper, freshly ground
- One teaspoon of natural sweetener (for example, honey) One teaspoon of powdered fennel seed (contains anethole and polymers, which help stomach issues) & 1/8 teaspoon fine sea salt (primarily used for flavor)

Directions:

1. Mix all powdered herbs in a bowl, except the fennel seed powder and sea salt. Then, gently heat the honey in a small saucepan until it is thinner and syrupier. Little by little, pour the honey into the powdered herbal mixture, constantly stirring until it can be molded into pea-shaped balls.
2. Roll these balls into the fennel seed powder and sea salt to create a coating. Take one 15 minutes before each meal.

Echinacea Remedy

Used for:

This remedy is perfect for canker sores.

Ingredients:

- Two tablespoons of sage tincture
- Two tablespoons of echinacea tincture
- Two tablespoons of lemon balm tincture

Directions:

1. Combine the three tinctures in a dropper bottle.
2. Use one dropper full of the mixture to swish around your mouth 2-3 times daily.

Chamomile Remedy

Used for:

The remedy is brilliant for clearing a stuffy nose. Repeat as needed.

Ingredients:

- Two handfuls of chamomile flowers, dried
- Ten chamomile tea bags (a relaxing, rejuvenating herb)
- Boiled water

Directions:

1. Boil 2 quarts of water, then add the dried chamomile flowers. Cover the pot and leave for 15 minutes beforeplacing it on a heating pad.
2. Place a towel over your head as you breathe in the steam by leaning over the pot; this will help unblock your sinuses.

Rosemary-Infused Oil

Used for:

Hair growth, mental clarity, pain reduction, the common cold.

You can use this infused oil for a hair mask, cooking, and in balm and salves.

Ingredients:

- Rosemary leaves
- Carrier oil (like olive oil)

Tools:

Quart jar Cheesecloth Glass bottles

Directions:

This method doesn't have specific measurements; it's okay to eyeball it.

1. Rinse your rosemary, making sure to dry completely. Put the herbs in a quart jar with 1-3 inches of space. For a multipurpose infusion, olive oil is a great choice. Fill the jar halfway with olive oil, leaving at least 1 inch of space between the herbs and the top of the jar. Close the lid tightly and shake well.
2. Set the jar on a sunny windowsill for three weeks, stirring every day. We've seen formulas that let the rosemary infuse for up to a month. Cover the jar with a paper bag if it's particularly hot outside. When

infusion time has passed, strain the oil through a cheesecloth into a cup or bowl. With a funnel, pour into clean glass bottles. Write "Rosemary oil with olive oil" and the date on the label. Store for up to a year in a dry, cold, dark location.

Directions for using dried rosemary:

Oil made using this method should not be ingested. An oil infusion with ground dried herbs and alcohol creates a potent mixture. You will need to measure out the ingredients. You'll need:

- 1-ounce rosemary, dried
- ½-ounce alcohol
- 8-ounces oil

Directions:

1. Grind your rosemary into a coarse powder. Don't pulverize it entirely into dust, or it will be hard to strain. Move the ground herbs into a clean jar. Pour in
½-ounce alcohol. Close the lid tightly and shake well. Wait for 24 hours.
2. Pour the herb/alcohol mixture into a blender or food processor. Start with about 8 ounces of your oil. You need enough oil to mix the herbs thoroughly. Blend for about 5 minutes.
3. Strain oil through a cheesecloth-lined, fine-mesh strainer into a bowl. Squeeze out the cheesecloth to get as much oil as possible. Funnel into glass dropper bottles and labels. Keep cold, dark, and dry for up to a year. For increased shelf stability, add a drop of vitamin E extract.

Calendula Salve

Used for:

Eases skin irritation, dried skin, eczema, and wound healing.

Calendula has antifungal, antibacterial, and anti-inflammatory properties. A salve made with this herb is excellent for chapped lips, dry hands, cuts, scrapes, and bruises.

Ingredients to make the calendula oil:
- Calendula flowers, dried
- Coconut oil
- Vitamin E oil & Ingredients to make the salve:
- 4-ounces calendula-infused oil
- ½-ounces chopped beeswax

Directions for the oil:

1. If your coconut oil is solid, warm it very gently until it becomes liquid.
2. Put dried calendula flowers in a glass jar (leaving about ¼ of it empty) and fill with oil to cover the flowers.
3. Label your jar. Shake the jar every two to three days and place it on a sunny windowsill. After at least three weeks, the oil will be thoroughly infused. More prolonged infusions provide a stronger oil. A dab of vitamin E oil extends its shelf life.

Directions for the salve:

1. In a double boiler, add your infused oil and beeswax.

2. Heat and stir so the beeswax melts and mixes smoothly with the oil. Remove from the heat and funnel into a glass jar or tin. Let the salve cool before closing the lid.
3. Label the container; also, remember to write down the date. Keep cold, dry, and dark. Don't scoop out with your finger when using the salve, as this increases the risk of contamination. Use a swab. When stored properly, this salve can last up to 3 years.

Tulsi-Chamomile Tea

It decreases cholesterol levels, reduces stress, lowers blood sugar, and helps with cold symptoms.

Tulsi, or holy basil, is high in antioxidants. Chamomile also has many medicinal benefits, including anti-inflammatory compounds. Together, they make a tea that can help ease cold symptoms and stress and improve your heart health.

Ingredients for fresh tea (makes five 1-cup servings):

- 5 cups water
- A handful of holy basil leaves, fresh (or 1 ½ tablespoon holy basil, dried)
- Two tablespoons of chamomile flowers, fresh (or one tablespoon of chamomile flowers, dried)
- Raw honey to taste

Directions:

1. Steep fresh leaves and flowers in hot water for 5-10 minutes. Strain and sweeten to taste.
2. You can also serve this tea with ice to make it chilly. You use dry leaves and flowers less because dry herbs have a more intense flavor.

COMMON DIY HERBAL RECIPES

Herbal Teas

Raspberry Tea

Serving size: 1 serving

Brewing time: 10 minutes

Ingredients:

- 1 cup water
- ¼ cup dried raspberry leaves
- ¼ cup dried lemongrass
- ½ cup dried chamomile flowers
- ½ cup dried orange peel

Directions:

1. Mix all the dried herbs listed above.
2. Boil water.
3. Add one teaspoon of tea mix to a cup.
4. Pour hot water over it. Cover and steep for 5-10 minutes. The longer the time, the more tannin is extracted.
5. Consume hot, cold, or iced.

Nutrition facts per serving: Calories: 40, Carbs: 12 g, Fat: 0 g, Protein 0 g, Sodium: 2 mg, Sugar: 0 g.

Hibiscus-Ginger Tea

Serving size: 4 cups

Brewing time: 15 minutes

Ingredients:

- 4 cups water
- 1 tablespoon of hibiscus leaves
- 1 tablespoon of grated fresh ginger
- 3-5 mint leaves

Directions:

1. Boil water in a pot.
2. Take hibiscus and ginger, then blend them in another pot.
3. Pour hot water over the tea mixture, cover, and steep for 10-12minutes.
4. The tea color will turn ruby red, then add mint leaves for fresh flavor.
5. Serve hot or cold.

Nutrition facts per serving: Calories: 1, Carbs: 1 g, Fat: 0 g, Protein: 0 g, Sodium: 1 mg, Sugar: 0 g.

Mint Tea

Serving size: 2 servings

Brewing time: 8 minutes

Ingredients:

- 2 cups water
- 15-20 fresh mint leaves
- Two lemon slices
- One teaspoon of honey (optional)

Directions:

1. In a teapot, boil the water.
2. Take the pan off the heat and toss all the mint leaves. Steep for 5 minutes with the lid on the pot. Increase the time for a strong flavor of mint.
3. Pour in a cup or glass.
4. Add honey and garnish with a lemon slice.
5. Enjoy hot or iced.

Nutrition facts per serving: Calories: 150, Carbs: 26 g, Fat: 5 g, Protein: 3 g, Sodium: 75 mg, Sugar: 15 g.

Sweet and Spicy Herb Tea

Serving size: 1 serving

Brewing time: 10 minutes

Ingredients:

- 1 cup water
- ½ tablespoon cloves
- 1 tablespoon of dried stevia
- ¼ cup cinnamon stick
- ¼ cup dried orange zest
- ¼ cup dried chamomile flowers
- ½ cup dried lemon verbena

Directions:

1. Make the blend and use one teaspoon of the tea mixture.
2. Boil the water and pour it over the tea mixture.
3. Cover the pot and steep for at least 5 minutes.
4. Strain into a cup and serve hot. Alternatively, pour over ice in the glass and serve cold.
5. Enjoy the sweet and spicy taste.

Nutrition facts per serving: Calories: 110, Carbs: 31 g, Fat: 3 g, Protein: 2 g, Sodium: 16 mg, Sugar: 1 g.

Basil Tea

Serving size: 1 serving

Brewing time: 5 minutes

Ingredients:

- 1 cup water & 1 teaspoon of basil leaves
- ¼ teaspoon dried ginger
- ½ teaspoon cinnamon powder
- 1 teaspoon of honey (optional)

Directions:

1. Boil the water and add the basil leaves, ginger, and cinnamon.
2. Steep it for 5 minutes.
3. Strain and add honey to improve the taste.
4. Pour in a cup and serve hot.

Nutrition facts per serving: Calories: 10, Carbs: 3 g,

Fat: 0 g, Protein: 0 g, Sodium: 1 mg, Sugar: 0 g.

Decoctions

Basil Decoction

Method:

1. Boil 2 – 3 tablespoons of basil leaves in a cup of water.
2. Steep for 10-15 minutes after covering with a lid.
3. Increase the number of basil leaves you use when making your decoction if you want the mixture to be more concentrated.
4. Put your hot decoction and strain it with a strainer or cheesecloth into an empty cup.
5. Thoroughly clean up the filter if used before storing it for later use.
6. Drink this hot herbal tea twice daily for best results.
7. You may want to include other ingredients in your decoction: mint leaves, rosemary, or lavender.
8. Also, note that rosemary can be used instead of basil for a more concentrated decoction.

German Chamomile Decoction

Method:

1. Boil 1 – 2 tablespoons of chamomile flowers in a cup of water.
2. Steep for 10-15 minutes after covering with a lid.
3. Take your hot chamomile decoction and strain it using a strainer or cheesecloth into an empty cup.
4. Thoroughly clean up the filter if used before storing it for later use.
5. Drink this hot herbal tea twice daily for best results.
6. You may want to include other ingredients in your

decoction: mint leaves, rosemary, or lavender.

7. Also, note that rosemary can be used instead of chamomile for a more concentrated decoction.

Chicory Decoction

Method:

1. Boil 1 – 2 tablespoons of chicory roots in a cup of water.
2. Steep for 10-15 minutes after covering with a lid.
3. Put your hot decoction and strain it with a strainer or cheesecloth into an empty cup.
4. Thoroughly clean up the filter if used before storing it for later use.
5. Drink this hot herbal tea twice daily for best results.
6. You may want to include other ingredients in your decoction: mint leaves, rosemary, or lavender.

Ginger Decoction

Method:

1. Boil 1 – 2 tablespoons of ginger in a cup of water.
2. Steep for 10-15 minutes after covering with a lid.
3. Put your hot decoction and strain it with a strainer or cheesecloth into an empty cup.
4. Thoroughly clean up the filter if used before storing it for later use.
5. Drink this hot herbal tea twice daily for best results.
6. You may want to include other ingredients in your decoction: mint leaves, rosemary, or lavender.

Ginkgo Berry Decoction

Method:

1. Boil 1 – 2 tablespoons of Ginkgo in a cup of water.
2. Steep for 10-15 minutes after covering with a lid.
3. Put your hot decoction and strain it with a strainer or cheesecloth into an empty cup.
4. Thoroughly clean up the filter if used before storing it for later use.
5. Drink this hot herbal tea twice daily for best results.
6. You may want to include other ingredients in your decoction: mint leaves, rosemary, or lavender.

Ginseng Decoction

Method:

1. Boil 1 – 2 tablespoons of Ginseng in a cup of water.
2. Steep for 10-15 minutes after covering with a lid.
3. Put your hot decoction and strain it with a strainer or cheesecloth into an empty cup.
4. Thoroughly clean up the filter if used before storing it for later use.
5. Drink this hot herbal tea twice daily for best results.
6. You may want to include other ingredients in your decoction: mint leaves, rosemary, or lavender.

Horsetail Decoction

Method:

1. Boil 1 – 2 tablespoons of horsetail in a cup of water.
2. Steep for 10-15 minutes after covering with a lid.
3. Put your hot decoction and strain it with a

strainer or cheesecloth into an empty cup.

4. Thoroughly clean up the filter if used before storing it for later use.
5. Drink this hot herbal tea twice daily for best results.
6. You may want to include other ingredients in your decoction: mint leaves, rosemary, or lavender.

Irish Moss Decoction

Method:

1. Boil 1 – 2 tablespoons of Irish moss in a cup of water.
2. Steep for 10-15 minutes after covering with a lid.
3. Put your hot decoction and strain it with a strainer or cheesecloth into an empty cup.
4. Thoroughly clean up the filter if used before storing it for later use.
5. Drink this hot herbal tea twice daily for best results.
6. You may want to include other ingredients in your decoction: mint leaves, rosemary, or lavender.

Popsicles

Ginger Mint Popsicles

Ingredients:

- One cup of coconut water or any fruit juice of your choice (if you are on a low-calorie diet, you can replace it with water).
- 2-inch ginger root, peeled and sliced into 1/4 pieces
- 4 to 6 fresh mint leaves

Process:

1. Add freshly sliced ginger and mint leaves to the blender. Pour in the fruit juice or coconut water. Blenduntil smooth.
2. Pour into popsicle molds and freeze overnight.

Cucumber and Herb Popsicles

Ingredients:

- 1 cup of fruit juice or coconut water
- Two cucumbers, peeled and sliced into 1/4 pieces
- 3-5 fresh mint leaves

Process:

1. Place the jar in the blender. Add in mint leaves and make sure that they are thoroughly blended.
2. Pour in the fruit juice or coconut water. Blend until smooth. Pour into popsicle molds and freeze overnight.

Fruit and Herb Popsicles

Ingredients:

- 1 cup of fruit juice or coconut water
- 2-inch piece of fresh ginger, peeled, sliced into 1/4 pieces
- 5 to 6 fresh mint leaves

Process:

1. Place the jar in the blender.
2. Add in mint leaves and ginger.
3. Make sure all ingredients are in proper condition.
4. Pour in the fruit juice or coconut water.
5. Blend until smooth. Pour into popsicle molds and freeze overnight.

Herbal Popsicles

Ingredients:

- 1Cup of fruit juice or coconut water
- 5 to 7 fresh mint leaves

Process:

1. Place the jar in the blender.
2. Add mint leaves and make sure that they are thoroughly blended.
3. Pour in the fruit juice or coconut water.
4. Blend until smooth.
5. Pour into popsicle molds and freeze overnight.

Cucumber and Mint Popsicles

Ingredients:

- 1 cup of fruit juice or coconut water
- One 2-inch piece of fresh ginger, peeled
- 5 to 7 mint leaves

Process:

1. Place the jar in the blender.
2. Add ginger and mint.
3. Make sure that they are thoroughly blended.
4. Pour in the fruit juice or coconut water.
5. Blend until smooth.
6. Pour into popsicle molds and freeze overnight.

Baths

Lavender Bath

Preparation:

1. Add 1 to 2 cups of dried lavender flower to your bathtub.
2. Boil a pot of water and add 1/2 cup of Epsom salt.
3. Pour the mixture into the bathtub, and then get into the tub after adding water.
4. Soak for 5 to 10 minutes.
5. Use with caution because the Epsom salt may irritate those who are sensitive to it.

Sage Bath

Preparation:

1. Place 1/4 cup of dried sage in your bathtub and add hot water.
2. Steep for 5 to 10 minutes before getting into the tub.
3. For extra effect, you can leave the herbs in the tub after your bath.
4. It is recommended not to use this herbal treatment if you are pregnant or breastfeeding because sage has some properties that can make youfeel like you're on an intense trip.

Rose Petal Bath

Preparation:

1. Place 8 to 10 organic rose petals into your bathtub.

2. Vitamin C is abundant in rose petals, which helps to brighten and soften the skin.
3. Steep the rose petals in hot water for 3 to 5 minutes before getting into the tub.
4. Rose glyceride is a substance in rose petals that can soothe the irritation and inflammation caused by eczema and acne.

Ginger Bath

Preparation:

Ginger is an essential element in improving your skin's health. The best ginger is fresh ginger, which can be added to your bath as a decoction or powder.

1. If you make the decoction, use two water parts for one part of ginger root.
2. For each person in the bath, add 1/2 cup of Epsom salt and 1 cup of fresh ginger root.
3. Use 3 to 4 cups of hot water for each person having the bath.
4. Steep in a pot for 5-10 minutes.
5. When ready to have the bath, use 1/2 cup of the mixture with the Epsom salt and add it to your bathwater.
6. Soak in warm water for 5 to 10 minutes before washing with cool water.

Do not use this herbal treatment if you have high blood pressure because ginger can increase blood pressure levels. Also, do not take this herbal bath if you are pregnant.

Breast Milk

Lemon Balm

Lemon balm has been found to help infants with colic, fussiness, and other digestive problems. Lemon balm has also been known to soothe infant fussiness and relieve cramps. In addition, studies have shown that lemon balm can help stimulate breast milk secretion and increase the nutrients in the milk of nursing mothers who take it.

Method:

1. Add 1/4 teaspoon of finely ground lemon balm powder or 2 to 3drops of lemon balm essential oil to 4 ounces of breastmilk.
2. Warm the breast milk either by the microwave or on the stove.
3. Serve your baby.
4. Repeat every two hours during the day and as needed for relief.
5. Do not use this herbal treatment when breastfeeding a preterm infant.

Chamomile

Chamomile is a common herbal remedy for treating children's colic, fever, and teething.

This plant is also known to help reduce swelling, soothe irritable newborns, and soothe fevers.

It can also be used for making herbal infant teas or tinctures.

Method:

1. Add 1/4 teaspoon of finely ground chamomile or 2 to 3 drops of chamomile essential oil to 4 ounces of breastmilk.
2. Warm the breast milk either by the microwave or on the stove.
3. Serve your baby.
4. Repeat every two hours during the day and as needed for relief.
5. Do not use this herbal treatment when breastfeeding a preterm infant.

Calendula

Calendula is also known as marigold. It can be used to make herbal teas for infants, or it can also be added to a bath in a bit of water. In addition, Calendula has strong anti-inflammatory properties.

Method:

1. Add 1/4 teaspoon of finely ground calendula or 2 to 3 drops of calendula essential oil to 4 ounces of breastmilk.
2. Warm the breast milk either by the microwave or on the stove.
3. Serve your baby.
4. Repeat every two hours during the day and as needed for relief.
5. Do not use this herbal treatment when breastfeeding a preterm infant.

Washcloths

Eyewash

Preparation:

1. Add a few drops of water into an eye spray bottle.
2. Fill the rest of the bottle with peppermint essential oil.
3. Use these eye drops to clean the eye area.
4. This is very good for people who suffer from dry eyes, as they can treat them with one quick and simple alternative. Refrigerate in an airtight container after each use to ensure potency.
5. The eyewash can also be used for other purposes, such as treating conjunctivitis, blepharitis, and other eye issues.

Tongue Wash

Preparation:

1. Fill the tongue spray bottle with a few droplets of water.
2. Fill the rest of the bottle with thyme essential oil.
3. Use this tongue spray to clean the area around the mouth, and you will feel a soothing sensation on your tongue.
4. This is an excellent treatment if your mouth is filled with bad breath and a cleansing of the inside of your mouth. It can be stored for two weeks in an airtight container after use.
5. The tongue wash can be used on other body parts such as the inner thigh area, groin area, armpit, and

any other areas that may need a light cleaning and soothing.

Armpit Wash

Preparation:

1. Fill the tongue spray bottle with a few droplets of water.
2. Fill the rest of the bottle with lavender essential oil.
3. Use this armpit spray to clean your armpits, and you will feel a soothing sensation on your skin.
4. This is very good for people who work in the construction field, as it will help remove odors from the body and develop an antibacterial treatment for skin infections. It can be stored for two weeks in an airtight container after use.
5. The armpit wash can also be used on other body areas, such as the groin area, inner thigh area, and back of the neck, to get a good cleaning.

Inner Thigh Wash

Preparation:

1. Fill the tongue spray bottle with a few droplets of water.
2. Fill the rest of the bottle with lavender essential oil.
3. Use this inner thigh spray to clean the area around your groin, making you feel a soothing sensation.
4. This is very good for sports people, as it will help remove perspiration and bacteria that may cause infections. In addition, it can create an antibacterial treatment for skin infections. It can be stored for two

weeks in an airtight container after use.

5. The inner thigh wash can be used on other areas such as the armpit, groin, inner wrist, and other indispensable areas.

Inner Wrist Wash

Preparation:

1. Fill the tongue spray bottle with a few droplets of water.
2. Fill the rest of the bottle with lavender essential oil.
3. Use this inner wrist spray to clean the area around your hand, making you feel a soothing sensation.
4. This is very good for people who work in the construction field, as it will help remove odors from the body and develop an antibacterial treatment for skin infections. It can be stored for two weeks in an airtight container after use.

Tinctures

Indigestion Tincture

Preparation:

1. Add one tablespoon of dried mint leaves to a half cup of water in a pot.
2. Bring it to a boil, turn off the stove, and let it steep and cool down for about 10 minutes.
3. Line the alembic with a cheesecloth, and then add mint mixture through it into your bottle of choice.
4. Now, screw the cap on firmly and store it in a cool and dark place for at least two weeks.

5. Take two spoonsful of tincture into the mouth, then swish it around to spread it evenly on your teeth, gums, and other parts of the mouth.
6. After that, you can take more tinctures depending on how well you feel after the first application.
7. You can also add the tincture to your food or juices.

Unlock Bactericidal Properties: Cough and Cold Tincture

Preparation:

1. Mix one tablespoon of chamomile with one cup of water in a pot.
2. Cook for about five minutes, then cover and set aside to cool for at least ten minutes.
3. Use 2-3 drops of tincture as needed for cough or cold.

Unlock Anti-inflammatory Properties: Painkiller Tincture

Preparation:

1. Mix one tablespoon of chamomile with two cups of water in a pot.
2. Boil the mixture for about five minutes, and then cover it until it is cooled for at least ten minutes.
3. Use 2-3 drops of tincture as needed for headaches, cramps, or other types of pain.

Infusions

Sore Throat Infusion

Preparation:

1. Bring two cups of water and one teaspoon of fresh ginger to a boil in a kettle.
2. Allow 10 minutes to steep after turning off the burner.
3. Use 1-2 teaspoons of the mixture as often as needed for sore throat pain relief.
4. People who regularly take this infusion have fewer cases of sore throat yearly because they have strong bacterial resistance.

Infusion of Sage

Preparation:

1. Pour two cups of water into a pot, add one ounce of sage leaves, and bring it to a boil.
2. Allow 10 minutes to step after turning off the burner.
3. Use 2-4 teaspoons of the mixture as often as needed for chest colds.
4. People who regularly take this infusion have fewer cases of sore throat yearly because they havestrong bacterial resistance.

Infusion of Fennel

Preparation:

1. Pour two cups of water into a pot, add one teaspoon

of fennel leaves and bring it to a boil.

2. Allow 10 minutes to steep after turning off the burner.
3. Use 1-2 teaspoons of the mixture as often as needed for cold, cough, and respiratory disorders.
4. People who regularly take this infusion have fewer cases of constipation yearly because they have strong bacterial resistance.

Infusion of Valerian

Preparation:

1. Pour two cups of water into a pot, add one teaspoon of fresh parsley flowers and bring it to a boil.
2. Allow 10 minutes to steep after turning off the burner.
3. Use 2-4 teaspoons with ½ teaspoon of valerian root for insomnia, anxiety, and nervousness.
4. People who regularly take this infusion have fewer cases of insomnia yearly because they have strong bacterial resistance.

Infusion of Yellow Dock Tea

Preparation:

1. Bring two cups of water and one teaspoon of fresh dandelion to a boil in a kettle.
2. Allow 10 minutes to steep after turning off the burner.
3. Use 1-2 teaspoons for liver disorders, skin problems, and urinary tract infections.
4. People who regularly take this infusion have fewer liver disorders and skin problems yearly because they have strong bacterial resistance.

Infusion of Dandelion Tea

Preparation:

Pour two cups of water into a pot, add one teaspoon of fresh dandelion leaves and bring it to a boil.

1. Allow 10 minutes to steep after turning off the burner.
2. Use 1-2 teaspoons for liver disorders, skin problems, and urinary tract infections.
3. People who regularly take this infusion have fewer cases of liver disorders and skin problems every year because they have strong bacterial resistance.

ELIXIRS OF LONG LIFE

Elixirs of long life are popular in Middle Eastern culture and have been mentioned as far back as 4000 BC. History mentions these elixirs being consumed by Egyptians, Incans, Assyrians, and

Mesopotamians. The elixir is an extract from the flower of the water lily plant(Nymphaea caerulea). It is not a plant that grows in the bottom of marshes and ponds but a tissue with roots.

The history behind this product is known to have medicinal effects on various possible diseases such as tumors, asthma, arthritis, kidney stones, heart disease, and diabetes. This medicine can also result in fewer wrinkles while retaining skin hydration throughout your life. The use of the elixir is even said to slow the aging process and give a more youthful appearance.

In the study of medicine, this flower extract is known as Pituri, also Lablab Purpureus, because of its resemblance. It grows in temperate zones. It is a native plant that includes several species that have medicinal qualities. These species are Lablab purpureus, Sesbania aculeata, and Dolichos lablab.

Extracts are made from either squeezing or grinding the flowers of this plant. Some prescribe to use of both processes for any medicinal properties to be amplified. The flower must be harvested before it blooms and its freshness has not expired. Some refer to this as "Lotus" and others as Nymphaea Caerulea. The extract is mixed with honey, wine, or water, and the product is ready for consumption. It is said that those who consume this elixir can live up to 300 years of age.

This elixir can also be used for thinning hair and other skin problems such as acne and dry skin. It also helps to relieve asthma and arthritis. Some even use it as a remedy for kidney stones and heart disease. Unfortunately, this book cannot explain how this product is made or what is in it for the reader because of the lack of evidence. So, instead, we have focused on the effect of consuming this elixir to solvevarious ailments we may have.

Middle Eastern cultures have consumed this elixir for thousands of years, and it has been mentioned in multiple historical volumes. It is also said that Cleopatra drank it every day and lived to be 72 years old; when Augustus Caesar killed her enemies, her age was recorded at 80 years old.

It is said that Empress Theodora was healed from the plague after drinking a mixture of this elixir and strong liquor. Her recovery made her famous worldwide. It's also used to treat cancer, tumors, and asthma. Cleopatra is also said to have used it as a remedy to stop balding and other skin diseases, including acne and eczema.

Cleopatra was also believed to have used the elixir every day so she could preserve her youthfulness and beauty. She took an extreme step by applying this elixir to her face, arms, neck, legs, bosom, thighs, stomach area, and buttocks. She would bathe twice a day to wash it off and reapply it. As the years went by, she used this elixir for 150 years.

This ancient medicine is still consumed today by those familiar with the elixir's properties. How? Asians make their version by extracting the flower of Nymphaea caerulea. They use fresh flowers and then add them to water in a bottle, where they simmer for over 16 hours. After that, they strain it through fabric and glass mats before consuming it. The Middle Eastern version can be purchased at various places around the world. Amazon, eBay, AliExpress, etc.

The flower extract can also be found in dry form, but fresh flowers are recommended. According to legends, this elixir was traditionally made by hand and may take up to a year to complete. Nowadays, extractors make it more efficient by using machines to speed the process up. However, this is a more cost-effective technique; many claims that the medicine's effect is less potent when prepared.

The elixir is consumed as a beverage in Middle Eastern cultures, where it has been sometimes deemed both sweet and sour. It is believed that consistent use of this elixir will result in a slower aging process; this is because people who take it daily don't need to eat or drink as much, and their bodies can get all the nutrients they need.

The drink is said by some to have health benefits that extend beyond the 300 years mentioned above. The extract contained within this elixir is said to have various colors, and no color means no medicinal benefit. The therapeutic effects of this extract have been verified through scientific tests. The plant's flower nutrients can be found in broccoli, cauliflower, cabbage, carrots, asparagus, and other vegetables such as zucchini and cucumber.

Extracts of plants are also used to create medicine, and its most common use is to treat heart disease and respiratory issues. Other uses involve the treatment of diabetes, fatigue, cancer, tumors, Alzheimer's disease, and other neural disorders. Unfortunately, although its benefits have proven to be medicinal, it is not sold as a cure-all for many ailments one could have.

Scientists in the medical field are still studying extracts from this plant to make it more effective when treating specific diseases. However, they do say that people who consume the elixir daily can enjoy a more youthful appearance throughout their lives.

5 HERBS TO HAVE A HEALTHYLONG LIFE

Live healthier than most other people. People who ate foods high in phytochemicals lived five years longer on average than those who didn't, according to a study published in the journal Nature in September 2016. They also enjoyed better quality lives. The study revealed that the chemicals came from something called "phytochemicals." These were primarily found in plants and were natural substances that prevented cell damage and cancer.

Along with eating healthy food (which contains lots of phytochemicals), you should also take herbs for their health benefits. Herbs have long been used to treat a variety of health problems. And because these substances are much more potent than regular foods, they are more likely to trigger a strong healing response in your body.

With that in mind, let's look at five herbs you can use to live a longer, healthier life.

Oregano

Oregano is a purple-flowered plant with olive-green leaves. It is related to mint, thyme, marjoram, basil, sage, and lavender. The leaves, both fresh and dried, are often used in cuisine. It's also used as a medication on occasion.

Fresh oregano herb and oregano oil are great additions to any dish. On a per ounce basis, it contains four times the antioxidant activity of blueberries! A single tablespoon of fresh oregano has the same number of antioxidants as a medium-sized apple.

Oregano oil also contains beta-caryophyllin, which helps to decrease inflammation.

Turmeric

Turmeric is a natural plant used as a spice in several dishes. It's an Indian plant with a long history. It is also known as curcumin, the spice's active component. Turmeric powder is yellow when used as a culinary spice.

According to research published in the American Journal of Cardiology, adding the spice turmeric extract to your meals reduces your risk of heart attack by 56%.

Plus, according to a 2012 research published in the Nutrition Research journal, turmeric improves cardiovascular health as much as aerobic exercise!

It has a "primary polyphenol" called "curcumin," which is crazy but real.

Turmeric/curcumin is also said to protect the brain, reduce inflammation, and aid cancer treatment.

Cloves

Cloves have a digestive system-supporting effect in all systems of traditional herbalism. They've also been utilized to promote a healthy immune and respiratory system due to their warming and digestion supporting qualities. The highly fragrant qualities of this dried flower bud and its "numbing" feeling are due to its high quantity of Eugenol essential oil.

The "cloves" spice is a lesser-known herb in the kitchen. However, this spice is prized in research laboratories for having the highest ORAC (Oxygen Radical Absorbance Capacity) score of any spice. Meaning? Cloves have the most antioxidants. Cloves also kill parasites, fungus, and bacteria in the intestine.

Ginseng

Ginseng is a slow-growing perennial plant belonging to the Panax genus in the Araliaceae family. In certain areas, the plant is also known as Ginnsuu.

The plant "ginseng" is said to have heart-protective properties. For example, using it in your cooking increases blood flow, which helps transport blood to the heart when oxygen levels are low.

Additionally, Ginseng's increased blood flow aids in the reduction of blood platelet stickiness, lowering your risk of blood clots.

Ginger

Ginger is a shrub with yellowish-green blooms and leafy stalks. The ginger spice originates from the plant's roots. Ginger is native to Asia's warmer regions, such as China, Japan, and India, but it is cultivated in South America and Africa. It is currently grown throughout the Middle East for medicinal and culinary purposes.

Geraniol is a cancer-fighting compound found in the plant "ginger."

In addition, ginger is an anti-inflammatory, making it suitable for your heart and avoiding blood clots.

This herb is said to help strengthen the immune system and guard against atherosclerosis.

CONCLUSION

Native American Indian medicine and herbal remedies were used to heal and prevent illness. An herbal remedy is a cure-all because it is made from plants that grow all around you. Herbs can be applied to

the skin, eaten as food, or drunk as medicine. Some are grown for health care, while others are for cooking or crafts.

The medicinal use of herbs goes back far into history across the globe. For example, ancient Greeks used them in everyday life and medical practice. At the same time, Eastern Europe and Asia have long histories of folk remedies often based on herbal treatments for stomach or respiratory sicknesses.

From the Middle Ages, people began to develop systematic theories about the medicinal properties of various plants. The ancient Greeks and Romans had developed herbal medicine, but it became more formalized and systematic for Western Europeans.

Herbalism spread from the Middle East to Europe for centuries. During these centuries, European physicians observed many plants with medicinal properties that they believed could cure illnesses. These medical observations were compiled into books by Arab merchants and scholars who also introduced many plants to Europe, including some new ones.

It is said that antique herbal medicine was concocted long

ago in ancient times. It originated from the knowledge of Greeks, Romans, and other civilizations and developed over time. These remedies were used to treat internal and external illnesses in ancient times.

Herbs were used as a way to heal wounds, skin conditions such as rashes or burns, and sicknesses of the body. Ancient herbs were often combined with other herbs in remedy recipes for serious illnesses because plants like aloe leaves contain acids that can help cleanse a person's blood. Other plants like ginger root contain enzymes that can aid digestion and metabolism. Ancient people realized these facts about plants and developed recipes to treat different issues in their bodies with particular herbs.

Antique herbal medicine recipes were not just used for people with acute and chronic diseases. They were also used for a wide range of ailments, including ones like fever and colds. In addition, people would use them to help treat illnesses requiring medicines from other substances, like plant extracts or roots; this is because herbal medicine was much cheaper than the medicines available then.

Ancient people used natural plants in the healing process to treat their disease while also using medicinal stones such as crystals to aid this journey. For example, plants were known in ancient times to be used for treating fever as a cure for it. In addition, they would use the plants to treat different diseases and illnesses.

Using ancient herbal remedies is still important today when the body suffers from an illness. Physicians like herbalists are needed to help sick people through their research and medical knowledge. While modern medicine has improved over time, there are still ways to keep herbs handy so that they can be used to treat specific ailments or illnesses before modern medicine can come into play. These herbs will help get rid of particular health issues as well as prevent them before they start.

www.ingramcontent.com/pod-product-compliance
Lightning Source LLC
Chambersburg PA
CBHW051518030726
47592CB00006B/2326